:60 SECOND

MIND/BODY REJUVENATION

:60 SECOND MIND/BODY REJUVENATION

Quick Tips to Achieve Inner Peace and Body Fitness

by
Dr. Curtis Turchin, D.C., M.A.

New Horizon Press
Far Hills, New Jersey

Curtis Turchin
    :60 Second Mind/Body Rejuvenation

Interior Design: Susan M. Sanderson

Thera-Cane diagrams and exercises reprinted by permission.

Library of Congress Catalog Card Number: 99-70156

ISBN: 0-88282-181-4
New Horizon Press

Manufactured in the U.S.A.

2004   2003   2002   2001   2000 / 5   4   3   2   1

AUTHOR'S NOTE

The material in this book is intended to provide new insights and a quick overview of methods and information now available and to raise awareness about natural alternatives. Prior to beginning any of the treatments described herein for mind and body rejuvenation, they should be discussed with a licensed health care practitioner. The author and publisher assume no responsibility for any adverse outcomes which derive from the use of any of these treatments in a program of self-care or under the care of a licensed practitioner.

The information in this book is based on Curtis Turchin's research and practice. Fictitious identities and names have been given to characters in this book in order to protect individual privacy, and some characters are composites.

TABLE OF CONTENTS

INTRODUCTION

:60 Second Affirmation:
"I enhance my health, I enhance my longevity."

Our evolution toward an upright posture has been a long process. Over the last half-million years, humans have become more erect and lost most elements of their former hunched, ape-like carriage. Likewise, the shape and size of the human spine has adapted to this upright posture.

Primitive people had little opportunity to sit. Because their lifestyle required continual wandering and foraging for food, they spent most of their days standing, walking, running, lying and occasionally squatting. Unlike modern man, they had no need to spend their day bent over a workstation or desk.

Today, the computer revolution has virtually eliminated the need for an employee to leave their seat. Many workers spend their days slumped in chairs, squinting at computer screens, bending their necks to cradle their telephone receivers or performing repetitive tasks in awkward positions, leaving little need or opportunity for standing or stretching.

Many of us sit for breakfast, sit in a car, subway or bus on the way to work, sit most of the day on the job and then after a stressful day at work, spend the evening slumped in front of the television set. One might think that this practice would make us all stress-free, relaxed individuals. Unfortunately, this is not the case. Sitting itself is stressful on the human spine. Add to this the slouched way most of us sit and the unnatural design of the average chair and the problem only worsens. In fact, research indicates that one of the greatest predictors of ill health and spinal degeneration is sitting for prolonged periods of time.

Unlike upright posture, the evolution of our diet came about much later. Our ancient ancestors were wanderers who foraged for food, subsisting primarily on wild fruits, vegetables and meats. As time passed, however, towns and cities were built around farms that grew wheat and raised cattle. Soon the most common meals consisted of meat, bread and dairy products. A low-fat diet high in vitamins and minerals was replaced by one high in fat and refined carbohydrates. Obesity became more common and people began to suffer more "civilized" diseases such as heart attacks, gout and cancer. Although farming and urban development made life easier and gave man more free time, it also sowed the seeds of many unhealthy living habits.

Thomas Edison, the developer of the electric lightbulb, may have been unaware of the profound impact of his invention. No longer required to stop work at sundown, or forced to relax and unwind as darkness fell, people could work all night if they wished, no longer constrained by the light and dark cycle. The rise of technology pulled people further from their primitive roots and instincts, allowing them the freedom to live without regard for natural forces.

To function in this high-tech world people rely on clocks, e-mail and cell phones. Our time is compartmentalized into forty or fifty hour work weeks that do not allow us to live in tune with our primitive intuition and instincts. The result is obesity, chronic illness, insomnia, depression and anxiety. Cancer and heart attacks continue to increase as experts peddle the latest fad diets and exercise programs. However, we need more than a quick fix. We need a coherent, integrated program that teaches body awareness, proper nutrition and exercise in a new way. The :60 Second Rejuvenation Strategy is the first system that deals with all of these problems by teaching healthy living habits drawn from science, evolution, history and anthropology.

PROVING THE REJUVENATION STRATEGY

The principles of the :60 Second Rejuvenation Strategy promote a long and healthy life. Although I have drawn most of my information from medical research, clinical studies, anthropology and history, there is one more source of valuable insight. If we study the world's oldest living people, we find secrets crucial to enhancing our own health and longevity.

The towering Caucasus Mountains and deep, rugged valleys between Russia, Turkey and Iran link the Black and Caspian Seas. Shoto Gogoghian, a well-known researcher of centenarians in the former Soviet Union, conducted revealing research on the habits of the people in the Caucasus Mountains. As they grew older, he discovered, they typically reduced their work schedules, but never retired. Rather than the rigid schedules common in most urban areas around the world today, their daily routines tended to follow a rhythm more like those of our primitive ancestors—one closely linked to the natural biological rhythm.

Most of these long-lived individuals exercised all day long, primarily walking, chopping wood or gathering food, and most of their diet consisted of vegetables, supplemented by fruits, nuts, grains, dairy products and meat. This diet is the foundation of the :60 *Second Rejuvenation Strategy* diet. It is also quite relevant to note that very few of these individuals suffered from back or neck pain, nor did they spend much time sitting. Most of their days were spent standing or walking, with only occasional breaks to sit or lie down.

Dr. Stephen Jewett, in his article, "Longevity and the Longevity Syndrome," found that, like the people of the Caucasus Mountains, many other long-lived people were moderate eaters who consumed very little fat and large amounts of protein, with a diet that consisted of mostly fruits, vegetables and lean meats. They used very little medication, rarely drank alcoholic beverages or smoked, were not prone to worrying and usually slept well. These behaviors are consistent with those advocated by the :60 *Second Rejuvenation Strategy*. Other studies tend to reach the same conclusions. Research clearly documents that healthy, long-lived people tend to exercise regularly, eat a diet high in fruits and vegetables and lean meats, sleep well and avoid the typical stresses of an urban lifestyle.

In another revealing document entitled "The Framingham Study," 19,000 Harvard graduates compared the thinnest with the most obese individuals. They found that the most obese individuals had the highest incidence of heart problems and kidney disease as well as diseases of other types. One must realize that the diet espoused by the :60 *Second Rejuvenation Strategy*, as well as many other of the most successful diets, teach the importance of eating large quantities of fresh fruits and vegetables supplemented by lean meats. This low-fat diet provides a wide variety of nutrients and promotes a lean and healthy body.

Adding to these insights is the work of Dr. Nathan Pritikin who began treating heart disease in the 1970s and espoused a low-fat diet, supplemented by regular vigorous exercise. Another well-known physician, Dr. Dean Ornish, also advocates a low-fat diet, emphasizing fruits and vegetables and recommending the stress reduction techniques of deep breathing, relaxation and vigorous exercise. These physicians have documented powerful health benefits from these diet programs.

The following chapters will educate you about body alignment, nutrition, exercise and your natural biorhythms. You will learn simple exercises and principles that require less than one minute to perform. No longer will you be required to memorize long formulas or follow tedious exercise regimens to be healthy. By tuning in to your deep feelings and intuition, you can quickly become happier and healthier.

There is no need to experiment with fad diets, nor is there any need to become involved in complex exercise programs. Studies of our ancient ancestors, as well as modern-day research into the components of a healthy lifestyle, are fairly conclusive. The results of these studies are the foundation for the "ten commandments" of the *:60 Second Rejuvenation Strategy*.

:60 SECOND REJUVENATION STRATEGY TEN COMMANDMENTS

1. Eat mostly fruits and vegetables.
2. Supplement your diet with occasional servings of lean meat, eggs, nuts, whole grains and low-fat dairy products.
3. Exercise on a regular basis.
4. Sleep well—seven or eight hours per night is the minimum required for the average individual.
5. Don't smoke.
6. Drink alcohol in moderation or avoid it completely.
7. Meditate or pray regularly.
8. Sit infrequently—less than two or three hours per day is best.
9. Practice the principles of proper body alignment and breathing.
10. Have fun! Life shouldn't be too serious.

PART 1

ENRICHING LIFE THROUGH :60 SECOND TECHNIQUES

Chapter 1

THE FIVE STRESS ZONES—
THE QUICK RELEASE SOLUTION

:60 Second Affirmation:
"I age slowly, I age gracefully."

Roberto came to the United States from Ecuador, put himself through college and graduated cum laude from the Wharton School of Business. After five years of hard work for a respected Wall Street investment firm, he had attained all the external ornaments of success. His fashionable country home, graced by a Ferrari, made him the hero of his rural Ecuadorian family. Yet his picturesque, abundant lifestyle suddenly crumbled.

Late nights with stockbroker friends drinking martinis and smoking fine Cuban cigars pulled him away from his wife and five-year-old daughter. He learned too late his wife could not accept his drinking nor his workaholic lifestyle. She filed for divorce and custody of their child. Roberto's life was shattered. Alone, without his family, he sank deeper into his self-destructive patterns. He gained forty pounds, began taking drugs, became a serious alcoholic, made impulsive stock deals and lost vast sums of money. A visit to his medical doctor for his yearly check-up revealed even more bad news. Roberto's blood pressure and cholesterol had soared to dangerous levels. He had also begun to suffer from chronic back pain, neck pain and incapacitating headaches.

We began working with the easiest problem first, Roberto's chronic back and neck pain. When I questioned him about his work environment, it was *obvious that he was continually hunched over his computer terminal. We adjusted his workstation and taught him to stretch his taut neck and back muscles.*

He soon realized that he was always tense. He began to utilize stress release techniques to help him relax. As the stress release techniques gave him more self-control, he began to regain control over his life and develop a better relationship with his ex-wife and daughter.

Most of us recognize that stress causes our muscles to tighten. We also acknowledge that slouching creates unattractive posture along with sore back, neck and shoulder muscles. However, we do not usually realize that the combination of stress, muscle tension and poor posture may create chronic illness. Sitting upright, rigid and tense, is not proper posture. For proper, or neutral posture, you must align your body and place your muscles in balance with each other. Otherwise, an illness can actually develop at the location of tension and stress.

Scientific research has documented that areas of stress, tension and chronically tight muscles lead to local inflammation and irritation. The inflammation, in turn, causes physical damage to the muscles, which can eventually heal with scar tissue. Diseased tissue and tight, sore muscles may then result from this chronic stress. When an area of the body is chronically weakened or irritated, it is more susceptible to the onset of arthritis, cancer, ulcers and other ailments.

The development of an ulcer is an excellent example of how the stomach may suffer damage from stress. Asthma, colitis, headaches, eyestrain and other illnesses may also be at least partly the result of stress and the poor posture it creates. In fact, disease due to stress is so common that many doctors feel that the primary cause of most illnesses may be stress and anxiety. Preventing stress and improving your posture are important in creating a foundation for radiant health.

Several scientific and religious texts describe areas of the body that are sensitive to stress and illness. These texts agree on five specific areas of the body that are prone to tension. This chapter is devoted to teaching you to rid yourself of stress and posture related problems in those five zones.

The following exercises are the ones we gave Roberto to control his stress. These stress release techniques are designed to help you localize and reduce tension in your five primary stress zones. Each section includes exercises and relaxation techniques you can use to improve the quality of your life.

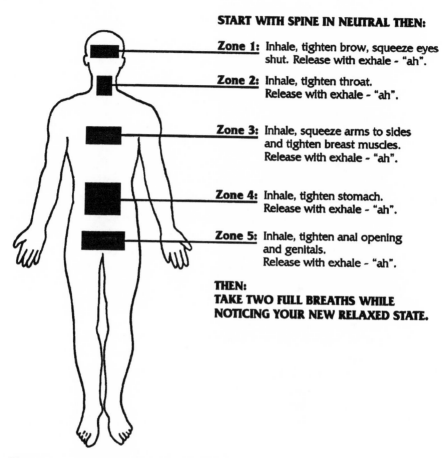

START WITH SPINE IN NEUTRAL THEN:

Zone 1: Inhale, tighten brow, squeeze eyes shut. Release with exhale - "ah".

Zone 2: Inhale, tighten throat. Release with exhale - "ah".

Zone 3: Inhale, squeeze arms to sides and tighten breast muscles. Release with exhale - "ah".

Zone 4: Inhale, tighten stomach. Release with exhale - "ah".

Zone 5: Inhale, tighten anal opening and genitals. Release with exhale - "ah".

THEN:
TAKE TWO FULL BREATHS WHILE NOTICING YOUR NEW RELAXED STATE.

Figure 1-1. Releasing the Five Stress Zones

Zone One

:60 Second Affirmation: "My forehead opens with clarity and light."
A common area for pain and tension, Zone One comprises the eyes, forehead and top of the head. Consider the average student anxiously taking a final exam or picture a parent late at night, slumped over tax forms. Both will repeatedly rub their eyes and forehead in an effort to ease their stress and strain. Squinting, blurry vision, headache and eye pain are all symptoms of strain in Zone One.

:60 Second Zone One Exercise: To release Zone One, relax all the muscles in your body. Inhale, tighten your brow and

squeeze your eyes shut forcefully while you silently count down from five to zero. When you get to zero, release all tension in your face and exhale, saying "ah." Take just a moment to enjoy the feeling of lightness and ease that this exercise generates. Let your body learn this new sensation as "normal."

Zone Two

:60 Second Affirmation: "Releasing the throat, my voice rings clear."
Zone Two is the throat. Stress can bring on a frog in your throat or the inability to speak clearly. Many of us under stress have experienced the need to "swallow our feelings." We may notice that sore throats, hoarseness, laryngitis and many other problems originate from tension and poor posture in the throat area. Matthias Alexander actually cured himself of a throat problem by improving his posture. He later developed the Alexander technique, the world's first systematic posture education program.

:60 Second Zone Two Exercise: Assume neutral spine posture. Close and tighten the muscles around your mouth, jaw and throat. This can be done by saying the "r-r-r" sound as if dragging the "r" in the word "rough." Inhale, tighten, count down from five to zero, then exhale with the "ah" sound and allow your throat to relax.

Zone Three

:60 Second Affirmation: "My chest and heart are open."
Zone Three is a band around the chest. The chest is the center of feelings. Some people have difficulty breathing when they "need to get something off their chests." The chest is also the container for the heart and the lungs. Symptoms of asthma and heart problems can increase in severity due to stress and tension in that area of the body. Hyperventilation, rapid heart beat and difficulty with deep breathing may all result from stress and tension locked in the chest area.

:60 Second Zone Three Exercise: Start in neutral with your arms hanging down. Take a deep breath and squeeze your arms firmly against your sides, tightening the chest and breast muscles, while silently counting down from five to zero. Exhale, relaxing all muscular tension. Take a few easy breaths, allowing the oxygen to bathe and nourish your body.

Zone Four

:60 Second Affirmation: "My belly softens and lightness fills me."
Zone Four contains the stomach and diaphragm. Chronic digestive problems are commonly associated with stress, anxiety and poor posture. For example, medical doctors and psychologists agree that stress is often the cause of stomach ulcers. A hiatal hernia occurs when stress draws the stomach up toward the chest, trapping it near the diaphragm. Slumping for hours in front of a computer terminal or the television set can also lead to a hiatal hernia.

> *:60 Second Zone Four Exercise:* To tighten your belly, it helps to pretend someone is about to punch you in the stomach. Now, inhale, tighten your stomach and hold your breath. Silently count down from five to zero, then exhale, releasing all tension.

Zone Five

:60 Second Affirmation: "I am open to life, I am open to love."
Zone Five is the lowest zone. It consists of the lower intestines, the anus and the sexual organs. Chronic diarrhea, constipation, bloating, hemorrhoids and sexual dysfunction can all result from stress and poor posture in this area of the body.

Most individuals experience a decrease in sexual ability or interest at some point in their lives. This is sometimes accompanied by poor digestion and tight muscles during times of increased stress. Many people have developed healthier sexual relationships by choosing the sexual postures that are right for them and avoiding positions that are uncomfortable.

> *:60 Second Zone Five Exercise:* Deeply inhale while tightening the sexual organs and anal opening. This exercise is similar to the medical exercise called the Kegel, described as a tightening of the muscles in the floor of the pelvis. Count down from five to zero; then exhale, releasing all tension in the anus, pelvic floor and sexual organs.

Stress is a common occurrence in all of our lives. It is associated with muscular tension and poor posture. By using our stress release techniques, you can eliminate anxiety and live a happier and healthier life.

THE FIVE STRESS ZONES:
ANATOMY AND PHYSIOLOGY

Each of the five stress zones has three separate layers. These are based upon the three primary embryological layers of tissue in the developing fetus. After the egg meets the sperm during conception, the resulting cell, called a zygote, begins to divide rapidly. After the cell implants in the uterine wall, it is called an embryo. The rapid cell division continues as three primary layers are formed. The three primary layers are the endoderm, mesoderm and ectoderm.

Layer One: Endoderm

The endoderm is the layer of cells which develop into your digestive tract. This layer of cells lines the mouth, throat, all of the internal organs and the anus. The energy level of an individual relies upon the efficiency of the digestive organs. In depression, the body's energy level is markedly lowered; there can be a loss of motivation, decreased appetite and shallow breathing.

The body is governed by two separate nervous systems, the sympathetic and parasympathetic. The sympathetic nervous system is responsible for the "fight or flight" response and prepares your body for action or survival. When you are engaged in a stressful situation, such as a violent and angry argument, being threatened or becoming overly fearful, your body slows or shuts down unnecessary functions to divert all energy to enable you to deal with the stressful situation and either fight or take flight. When your sympathetic nervous system is in control, for example, your heart rate increases while your digestive and sexual functions decrease. On the contrary, when the parasympathetic nervous system is activated, your body systems are brought back to normal levels of functioning; your heart rate is lowered, sexual energy rises and the digestion of food is facilitated. This parasympathetic state is one of deep calm and relaxation. Learning how to stand your ground, flee a dangerous situation or be angry uses your sympathetic nervous system. Learning how to relax, be sexual or be playful requires activation of the parasympathetic system.

The *:60 Second Rejuvenation Strategy* teaches you how to balance these two parts of your nervous system.

Layer Two: Mesoderm

The middle layer of the embryo eventually develops into bones, muscles, blood vessels and the heart. It is a system designed for movement and activity. Muscle tone can be unbalanced in two possible directions. Increased tone is created through an excess of muscle tension—more than is required for a particular action. The muscles feel hard, tense, spastic or rigid. Decreased tone results from a deficiency in muscle power—less than is required for a specific action. The muscles in this state feel soft, spongy, sluggish and unresponsive. To develop a healthy mind and body, you need to be able to increase and decrease your muscle tone. Physical activity and exercise requires increased tone, whereas sleep and rest require decreased tone.

The exercises in the *:60 Second Rejuvenation Strategy* teach you to balance your muscular tone. To be healthy and well grounded requires the ability to subconsciously shift between these two states of muscle tone—recruiting strength for vigorous physical activity and then turning on muscular relaxation to rest.

Layer Three: Ectoderm

The third cellular layer is the outermost layer, called the ectoderm. It includes all of the nerve tissue in the body, especially the sensory organs, spinal cord, nerves and skin. Skin is not only protection. Intricately tied to your nervous system, it also helps gather and integrate information about the world around you. The nervous system also coordinates information from all three embryological layers. It helps you to perceive sensation from your gut and then activates your muscles with a response. Through your sight, hearing, smell, taste and sense of touch, you are able to receive information from your environment. You accept this information and feed it into your spinal cord, sending it to your brain for processing. Your ectoderm, or nervous system, can be imbalanced, causing you to be overly sensitive or insensitive to stimuli.

The overly sensitive individual is easily excitable and stressed. The insensitive person tries to avoid information. The sensitive person can be easily threatened, thin-skinned and easily agitated. The insensitive person is thick-skinned and well defended. Neither extreme is optimal; thus, one goal of the *:60 Second Rejuvenation Strategy* is to help you integrate the three layers of each of your five stress zones and find a healthy balance. Proper breathing is an important part of the *:60 Second Rejuvenation Strategy* because it helps to integrate all three layers of your five stress zones. Relaxed, easy breathing restores the body's natural, physiological balance, thereby improving the function of your nervous system, muscles and digestive organs.

BLOCKING OUR FEELINGS,
BLOCKING OUR POWER

Slouching for a long period of time or feeling stressed results in tight muscles or knots, a natural response to emotional and physical tension that can occur everywhere in the body. Muscles require the ability to regularly contract and relax to be healthy. If muscles remain in a state of chronic contraction, muscular damage occurs. This contraction of muscles leads to swelling and inflammation, which always heals with fibrous scar tissue. This scar tissue forms tiny muscular blocks that restrict motion, reduce movements, stifle breathing and give rise to feelings of anxiety.

Muscular blocks can occur in or around any of your five stress zones. By learning the breathing and relaxation exercises taught in the *:60 Second Rejuvenation Strategy*, you can break down these muscular blocks. Because your mind and body influence one another, learning physical exercises and relaxation techniques will release these muscular restrictions.

By integrating your mind and body through breathing, meditation and exercise, you can release all five stress zones. Natural breathing and a flexible body form the basis for a calm mind and overall spiritual, mental and physical health.

:60 SECOND STRESS REDUCTION SUMMARY

- Muscle tension and poor posture may create chronic illness.
- Gain self-control; learn to relax.
- The five primary stress zones are: forehead, throat, chest, abdomen and pelvis.
- Practice the five stress release techniques several times a day.
- Help your body learn these new healthy sensations as normal.
- Each of the five stress zones has three separate layers: endoderm, mesoderm and ectoderm.
- Proper breathing is a crucial part of the *:60 Second Rejuvenation Strategy* because it helps to integrate all of your five stress zones.
- By integrating your mind and body through natural breathing, you can control the conscious and unconscious parts of you—your five stress zones and your three layers.

Chapter 2

ALIGNING EFFORTLESSLY—
EXERCISES FOR NATURAL POSTURE

:60 Second Affirmation:
"I align my body, I align my spirit."

Melanie worked for a large aerospace corporation in Silicon Valley. She came to me complaining of chronic lower back pain. She had previously seen her medical doctor, an orthopedic surgeon, a neurologist and two physical therapists, but no one could solve the dilemma of her back pain. Constant use of anti-inflammatories had caused a bleeding ulcer, forcing her to deal with the pain—without medication.

Melanie had the classic signs of a bulging lumbar disk. She told me that she had spent eight hours a day sitting at her computer for the last thirty years and never noticed how poor her posture was. Then, without any warning, she developed chronic lower back pain that persisted for two years prior to her coming to my office. Melanie was exercising on a regular basis, performing both stretching and strengthening, and she even iced her back twice a day. She told me I was her last hope. I showed Melanie the neutral spine posture and explained that she was to practice finding the neutral sitting and standing positions throughout her work day. She agreed to give it a try. After all, nothing else had worked, and she was desperate. Six months later, Melanie returned to my office for a check-up and reported that her back pain had been drastically reduced.

YOUR SPINE

Some of the most common and most easily remedied health problems are those associated with back pain. Yet most people believe they are helpless against these ailments. The human spine is composed of three basic curves: the cervical curve in the neck, the thoracic curve in the middle back and the lumbar curve in the lower back. Designed so that each arch sits on top of the one below, slouching distorts the relationship of these arches. The most effective method of preventing the pain associated with spinal stress is to maintain these arches in their most natural position. Called the *neutral spine posture*, this position allows each arch to be in its optimal position.

The spine is composed of thirty-three vertebrae—twenty-four separate and nine fused. Each vertebra is a block made of bone. When there is excessive stress placed upon these vertebrae, they will actually produce more bone at the areas of stress to protect and stabilize the region. The extra, unwanted bone, called degenerative arthritis, is not the same as rheumatoid arthritis or osteoarthritis, which causes crooked and swollen fingers. Rheumatoid arthritis and osteoarthritis are hereditary diseases, while degenerative arthritis of the spine results from wear and tear, caused by poor posture or trauma to the spine.

Above and below each vertebra are disks and joints. When you are in a neutral spine posture, each disk and joint is in an ideal position, resting effortlessly, floating in relationship to the adjacent vertebra. However, when you bend, these joints and disks become stretched.

The disks serve as pads, which separate each vertebra. Each disk has fluid in the center, called the nucleus. This nucleus is in the shape of a ball of jelly that allows the disk to roll as if it were on a ball bearing. Holding these balls of jelly in place are fibrous bands of tissue, called annular fibers. These fibers act like scotch tape that is wound around the ball of jelly, keeping it in correct position.

If you put stress on a disk, these annular fibers begin to tear, allowing small amounts of jelly from the nucleus to leak out. If the fibers are torn completely, the disk will rupture and much more jelly will leak out, resulting in what is commonly referred to as a herniated disk. This is a very serious problem that could require medical treatment or even surgery. Proper posture allows the annular fibers to hold the nucleus in its perfectly centered neutral position at the center of the disk. Maintaining proper posture reduces the possibility of ever rupturing a disk.

At the top and bottom of each vertebra, just behind the disks, are the joints. Each joint is very much like a joint in your finger. On each side of the joint are ligaments which act like rubber bands that are attached to both ends of each joint to keep the structures together. When you slump or twist in contorted positions, ligaments become overstretched and may tear. If they tear, they become inflamed and heal up with fibrous scar tissue or calcium that eventually leads to degenerative arthritis. By using optimal posture and keeping your spine in the neutral position, you will slow down this process and eliminate the possibility of serious degeneration.

Avoiding trauma will also help to prevent degenerative arthritis. Assuming you are a fairly careful individual and avoid high-risk activities, it is unlikely that you will suffer significant spinal injury. Those engaging in high-risk activities such as rock climbing, motorcycle racing or hang-gliding typically suffer significant trauma to the spine. There are, however some types of trauma which are unavoidable. For example, whiplash sustained in a car accident or a serious slip-and-fall in the bathtub can cause minor damage to the spine. However, the majority of cases of degenerative arthritis are not caused by these small injuries. Rather, they are caused by the repetitive damage of poor posture. Understanding how to hold your body in a relaxed, neutral position will help prevent degenerative arthritis.

PROPER POSTURE

Proper posture is an essential element of a healthy, stress-free lifestyle, yet very few people use proper body mechanics. Proper posture is rarely taught in schools and is never taught by doctors. Even the average chiropractor or physical therapist rarely instructs their patients in the tenets of proper posture. If proper body alignment is so important, why is it so rarely taught? The reason is simple.

Proper posture has always been believed to be a static and rigid position. Standing straight and looking tall has always been more important than feeling good. This is the absurdity of old-fashioned and even most modern posture education. This book attempts to change these rigid concepts into easy, comfortable and logical exercises. Try the following exercises to find your neutral position.

:60 Second Hand Exercise

Start by finding the neutral position of your hand. Place your hand into a fist, as if you were going to punch a punching bag. This is the extreme closed position of your hand. Next, open your hand as far as it will possibly go. This is the extreme open position. Now, extend your fingers so you hold your hand completely straight or flat. This straight or flat position of your hand is very similar to the position of your spine which might mimic the *proper posture*. Notice that everything is straight. It is the midway point between the flexed position (a fist) and the extended position (hand maximally opened). Neither of these is the neutral or natural position of your hand, however. Now, try the following:

Place your hand at your side or in your lap in its most relaxed state. Leaving your hand in this most relaxed state, elevate it in front of your face so you can look at it. Notice that your hand is in a slightly flexed or cupped position. It is not flexed into a fist nor is it extended as far as it will go. Also, it is not in its most rigid or straight position. This relaxed position of your hand is called *neutral*. It is the *natural resting position* of your hand. Notice that when your hand is in this neutral position, hanging at your side, it is almost straight. But, it is far more comfortable than a rigid, straight position. This is the ideal, natural or neutral position of your hand.

Practice finding the neutral or natural position for your spine while sitting, standing and lying down by using the following exercises.

:60 Second Lower Back: Sitting Exercise

Sit in a chair or on a stool in an upright position. If you are in a chair, be certain that you are not touching the back of the chair.

Notice that you are sitting on two bones. These two bones are called your *ischial tuberosities*. They are commonly referred to as your *sits bones* because they are the bones that form the very bottom of your buttocks and provide the foundation for sitting. Begin by rounding your lower back, slightly slumping forward. Next, return to the upright position. Now, position yourself in a rigid upright position by arching your lower back forward and leaning your shoulders and neck back slightly. Finally, return to the neutral position, the position in between these two extremes.

Practice this a few times. First, sit in an upright position between the two extreme positions. Then, gently round your back and flex forward, and then gently arch your back so that you slightly lean backwards. Lastly, return to the most comfortable position for your lower back in between these two extremes. This is the neutral, or natural position for your lower back.

:60 Second Lower Back: Laying Exercise

Lie down on the floor, or bed. Notice that your lower back naturally finds its most comfortable position. Next, flatten your back against the bed or floor. Flattening your back is easier if you tighten your stomach muscles at the same time. Then, relax the stomach muscles once again and return to the neutral position. Now, perform the opposite. Arch your back, increasing the lower back curvature, elevating your abdomen toward the ceiling. Now, return to the neutral or natural low back position.

Practice this a few times, flattening your back against the bed or floor, then arching your back elevating it maximally and finally relaxing your back to find the neutral or natural lower back position. Notice that in this neutral position, your back is in a state of maximal relaxation with the joints in their position of natural alignment. You might find that the natural position for you is slightly flattened or slightly arched.

This neutral or natural position may change with age and with time. However, every lower back has its own unique natural or neutral position, depending upon its shape, your level of health and your level of fitness. For example, pregnant women often report that the shape of their lower back changes as the pregnancy progresses. Therefore, they would find that the natural or neutral position would change over time. This is a natural response to the changing weight placed upon the spine.

MASTER THE POSITIONS

You have now learned the natural position of your hand and the natural position of your lower back while sitting and lying down. You may stop here and proceed with other chapters to build upon the concepts which we have developed using the neutral position of the hand and lower back, or you may proceed to learn how to hold all of your body in the neutral position. If you move to the other chapters, return here from time to time until you have mastered all of the positions.

The Lower Back: Standing Exercise

Stand with your feet approximately hip width apart. This is easiest to perform if your knees are also in the neutral position. Place your knees in an unlocked, flexible position. Bend your knees just slightly, as if you were trying to squat. Return your knees to the original position. Next, place your knees in the other extreme by locking them backwards–you will feel resistance to this position. Now, find the neutral or natural position of your knees by placing them between the slightly bent position and the locked rearward position. This is the neutral position for your knees.

In the standing position, try to find your neutral or natural low back position. As in the previous exercise, move your lower back into the two extreme positions–arched then curved. As you arch your back, notice that this causes you to pouch your stomach out slightly. Next, return to the neutral position. Then, flatten your back while tightening your stomach muscles. These are the two extreme postures of your lower back in the standing position. Just as with sitting and lying, you can find your neutral low back position while standing.

The Neck

Finding the neutral position of the head and neck is very easy if you will think about how a pigeon walks. Visualize a pigeon moving its head forward and back as it walks while you perform the neck exercise.

In the sitting or standing position, gently tuck your chin towards your chest while pulling your head back. Another image might be the head position of a soldier at rigid attention—the head is retracted maximally. Now, relax the muscles in your neck and let your chin move slightly forward. Then, jut your chin out, thrusting your head forward. Then, return to the natural or neutral position.

Again, practice moving your head into the neutral or relaxed position. Then, thrust your head forward, return to neutral and tuck your chin, thrusting your head backward. Always return to the neutral position.

If you have trouble with this or if you suffer from neck problems, it may be important for you to learn more about holding your head in this neutral position. If so, continue with the more advanced head and neck position exercises below. Otherwise, you may move on to the section on the shoulders and middle back.

NOTE: If you experience moderate to severe pain while trying to do these simple motions, it may be an indication that one or more of the vertebrae in your back is stiff. In this case, you may consider seeing a licensed physical therapist, doctor or chiropractor for treatment.

:60 Second More Advanced Neck Exercises

Many people are unaware that they continually twist or tilt their heads in positions that place pressure on the vertebrae and muscles in the neck. To learn more about relieving this tension, try the following exercises standing in front of a mirror.

While looking straight forward, try to position your head so that it is properly balanced on top of your shoulders. Make sure that your ears are approximately the same distance from the top of your shoulders. Now, bend your left ear toward your left shoulder and return to the neutral position. Then, bend your right ear toward your right shoulder, followed by returning to the upright or neutral position. Spend a few seconds in this neutral position, finding the comfortable and most balanced position for your head. Although ideally both ears should be an equal distance from your shoulders, you should be more concerned about your neck feeling comfortable. Never force symmetry upon your body, because it is more important to find the comfortable neutral position than to be perfectly symmetrical and upright.

Now, carefully rotate your head as far as possible to the right, and then return to neutral. Then rotate your head as far as possible to the left, and return to neutral. You might try this with your eyes closed. If you can rotate your head to both sides with your eyes closed and then return to the neutral position, you are doing very well. If you experience pain doing this motion, do not force your neck.

:60 Second Shoulder and Middle Back Exercise

In the sitting or standing position, find your neutral or most relaxed position. Now, round your shoulders forward, as if you were trying to touch your shoulders in front of your chest. Then, return to the neutral or relaxed position. Next, draw your shoulder blades backwards, trying to pinch them together in the middle of your back. Again, return to the natural or neutral position. Repeat this a few times until you have mastered this neutral position of the shoulders and middle back.

Practicing The Neutral Positions

You have now learned the neutral position of your hands, lower back, middle back and neck. Practice finding these positions throughout the day. You can practice these positions while you are sitting or standing on the subway. Practice them in your car during traffic jams, when standing in line at the bank, supermarket or movie theater. Or, practice them while lying in bed when you wake up in the morning or prior to going to sleep. Obviously, it may be most important to practice the positions that are most common to your lifestyle. For example, if you sit most of time at work, practice these techniques while at your desk. Whether you are sitting at the computer, talking on the telephone or in a business meeting, you may use these posture concepts very gently, without being noticed. Continue to return to these exercises, especially the lower back movements, when you are sitting for long periods of time.

If you sit most of the day, you should also get up every twenty to thirty minutes and walk around for :60 seconds prior to returning to the seated position. This will ensure that you remove the stress on your lower back regularly and maintain good blood circulation all day long. Good circulation is essential for the health of your heart and lungs. And by learning to maintain neutral posture, you are living in a state that is more natural and based upon deep, primitive instincts.

PREVENTION IS THE BEST CURE

Proper alignment is the most effective way to prevent spinal stress, spinal degeneration, pain and injury. By understanding how to maintain the neutral spine position that is your body's natural posture, you will feel that sitting, standing and moving are effortless. This feeling of free movement and comfort can be the foundation for your emotional, physical and spiritual well-being. You will only feel as young as your spine is healthy. Feelings of joy, heightened awareness and pleasure that result from feeling comfortable will help you experience the benefits of the natural posture principle.

:60 SECOND NEUTRAL POSTURE SUMMARY

- With proper posture, it is almost impossible to rupture a disk.
- Ligaments may become overstretched and tear as a result of poor posture, causing inflammation, fibrous scar tissue or calcium build-up.
- Rheumatoid arthritis and osteoarthritis are hereditary diseases; degenerative arthritis results from the wear and tear caused by poor posture or trauma.
- Avoiding trauma and poor posture will prevent or slow down the process of degenerative arthritis.
- A pain-free spine in proper alignment is the foundation for your emotional, physical and spiritual health and well-being.
- Maintaining natural, fluid posture will help you to tune in to primitive instincts and intuition.
- Proper posture is an essential element of a stress-free lifestyle; it is not a static and rigid position.
- Master the neutral or natural positions for your hands, lower back, neck, shoulders and middle back.
- Practice finding these positions several times a day, any time of day.
- Return to these exercises often, especially the lower back movements, when you sit for long periods of time.
- Stand up every twenty to thirty minutes or so and walk around for at least :60 seconds if you sit most of the day.

Chapter 3

BREATHING AWAY STRESS— STOP HOLDING YOUR BREATH

:60 Second Affirmation:
"My body is a foundation of
emotional, physical and spiritual well-being."

Linda had overcome an abusive childhood, punctuated by bouts of depression. Establishing healthy interpersonal relationships and a happy marriage while developing a successful career as a marketing executive was a serious challenge, but she achieved contentment. Her newfound emotional well-being was interrupted by a tragic motorcycle accident. While riding on the back of her husband's motorcycle, traveling at approximately sixty miles per hour, they struck a large boulder which had rolled off the hillside onto the freeway below. She and her husband became projectiles, hurtling through the air and then falling frightfully to earth. They were airlifted by helicopter to the nearest trauma center. Her husband suffered a serious concussion and Linda suffered multiple fractures to her neck, shoulder and forearm.

After three years of physical rehabilitation, Linda was sent to me by her orthopedic specialist. She still complained of chronic pain throughout her neck, back and arm. Two months of gentle soft tissue therapy yielded significant improvement, however she still suffered from some back and neck pain. She asked if she could perform her stretches more vigorously. I cautioned her against aggressive exercise, knowing it could aggravate her condition. But I encouraged her to slowly increase the range of her stretching exercises, while paying close attention to her symptoms to prevent further injury.

After two weeks of deeper stretching, she reported that whenever she stretched her neck she felt like crying. I explained to her that we associate our feelings at the time of the injury with the physical trauma. Our will to survive can often require us to repress these intense emotions while we struggle to rehabilitate ourselves. Years of psychotherapy still may not trigger the release of these feelings unless there is some movement or touch to trigger the memory of the physical experience. I encouraged her to continue stretching and to allow her emotions to flow freely.

Like many survivors of physical trauma and abuse, she was a very anxious, shallow breather. I worked with her during our next session on the belly-chest-exhale technique and encouraged her to use it while she was stretching and to consciously breathe deeply every time she was aware of her shallow breathing. I told her that, while exercising, each exhalation should include a "sigh" or some other sound that reflected the emotional or physical pain that she experienced. She told me that stretching and strengthening exercises would occasionally bring up old, trapped memories from her childhood and teenage years. It was with Linda that I made a unique discovery. I learned that natural breathing and posture exercises, combined with strengthening and stretching exercises, could bring up deep-seated feelings. It appeared that breathing and exercise could be a deep pathway into the soul.

BREATH: THE MISSING LINK

Integrating your mind and body is no easy task. Our ancestors were not bombarded by traffic jams, violent video games and the stress of a fifty-hour work week. Primitive man had periods of great difficulty due to harsh weather, famine, disease and the potential threat of wild animals and hostile invaders. However, these events were naturally interspersed with the rhythm of relaxation. Our lives, on the other hand, have become mechanical and regimented, forcing us to cope without time for rest and reflection.

This increased psychological stress causes us to constrict all of our stress zones. We have adapted to these modern stresses by taking on huge amounts of responsibility and abandoning awareness of our deep primitive, intuitive selves. While you cannot physically contact your organs, touch your soul or easily modify your nervous system, proper breathing provides one way of organizing and balancing your entire body. Natural breathing is the connection that unifies all of these disparate areas.

Breathing is one of the few functions of the human body that can easily be conscious or unconscious. You can go about your day, running errands, totally unaware of the rhythm of your breathing. Although breathing patterns are usually unconscious, you do have the ability to control them. Your breathing reflects your emotional and physical state at any point in time and is therefore an important part of healthy living. During times of great stress or heavy physical exercise, you become highly aware of how you are breathing. But these periods of awareness are rare. People are usually oblivious to the ebb and flow of respiration. By learning natural breathing, you are able to integrate and balance your metabolism by improving the function of your nerves, digestive tract and muscular system. That is why it is common to say you are *centered* when you are connected to the rhythm of your breathing. Being centered implies that your central physiological and emotional processes are functioning optimally.

Breathing Exercise

Very few people realize that breathing and heart rate are intimately related. Between your rib cage and stomach is your diaphragm. This sheet of tissue forms a dome between your rib cage and your gut. It is connected through other anatomical structures to your stomach and to your heart. When your breathing is relaxed and fluid, it will regulate your heart rate.

Inhale and exhale a few times, and notice how you breathe. Most of us breathe first into our bellies and then into our chest. Therefore, your belly will inflate before your chest. When you exhale, you should exhale through the chest and belly simultaneously.

Although inhaling first into your belly and then into your chest comes naturally, most of us do not think about how we breathe. In order to utilize breathing as a means of stress reduction and relaxation, it is important to be conscious of how we breathe. We can raise our awareness of our natural breathing by concentrating on it through the following simple exercise. Close your eyes and try breathing first into your belly, then into your chest and then exhaling. Now, pay attention to the amount of time between your inhale and your exhale. There should be a brief pause between your inhale and your exhale and a longer pause between your exhale and your inhale.

Try the following as you breathe: Inhale and silently say, "belly, chest." After a brief pause then silently say, "exhale, rest." Although there is a slight pause between your inhalation and your exhalation, the longer pause occurs after you have exhaled air, prior to breathing in again. Be certain that you rest between your exhale and inhale. Remember that anxiety can cause a racing heartbeat and difficulty breathing. Natural breathing will help you control high blood pressure and lung problems.

When practicing this exercise, sit in a comfortable position using the *:60 Second Rejuvenation Strategy* posture exercise if you're uncertain about how to position your body in its most natural state. Also try closing your eyes and repeating silently, "belly, chest; exhale, rest." Repeat this phrase as you slowly breathe, focusing only on the rhythm of your breath. This exercise is what we refer to as the *belly-chest-exhale technique.*

REDUCING YOUR STRESS

If you feel stress at any point during your day, use this brief :60 second breathing exercise to reduce your stress and synchronize the relationship between your breathing and your heart. This exercise can be done any time and in any place, whether you're at work, on the subway or stuck in traffic. There is always time to take a few breaths and relax.

If this becomes second nature, you might try using a different phrase, such as an affirmation, a mantra or a peaceful visualization. Thinking to yourself a phrase such as, "Breathing in I clear my mind; breathing out I rest," or visualizing a relaxing image may help you breathe in a more relaxed and regular fashion.

:60 Second Aligning Body and Emotions Strategies

It is possible to take the :60 Second Rejuvenation Strategy's breathing exercises one step further. Although this is no substitute for psychotherapy, it will help you to alleviate emotional stress, decrease body tension and relieve yourself of unwanted, uncomfortable feelings.

While dramatic, emotional outbursts might not be appropriate during your local aerobics or yoga class, emotional release through stretching can be performed in the privacy of your own home or with a therapist. When performing the exercises described in the :60 Second Rejuvenation Strategy or performing other stretching exercises, follow these suggestions:

1. Stretch in a comfortable place. A mat on a carpeted floor or a firm mattress are ideal.
2. Breathe using the belly-chest-exhale technique.
3. Exhale with a sigh or a sound that reflects your current feelings.
4. Allow emotions to surface, but do not force them in any way.
5. Do not force yourself to express a feeling, but do not stifle a feeling when you sense it arising.
6. If you find feelings difficult to access or if they frighten you, seek professional help. Psychotherapists, religious counselors and doctors are all sources of practical help should you feel the need.

ADVANCED :60 SECOND TECHNIQUES

If you find that breathing naturally and making sounds while stretching relieves stress and tension, you might want to go even deeper. One technique to provoke the release of deeper feelings is reverse breathing, or breathing in the opposite order of the belly-chest-exhale technique. Try breathing first into your chest, then into your belly, followed by an exhale with a sigh. Perform this reverse breathing pattern a few times whenever you want to release your deepest feelings. Always follow reverse breathing with the natural breathing cycle, using the belly-chest-exhale technique.

:60 Second Relax Away Stress Exercise: Lie on your back with your arms at your sides, knees bent and feet flat on the floor. Place your left hand on your heart and your right hand just below your navel. Breathe naturally, following the belly-chest-exhale technique, and then pause before breathing in again. To relax further, inhale and exhale slowly and quietly through your nose. Keep your jaw relaxed with your mouth closed. Now, move through your five stress zones by gently tightening the muscles in each zone, followed by five to ten gentle breaths. Begin by contracting your anal sphincter muscle, then take a deep breath and exhale, allowing the sphincter muscle to open, widen and relax. This should be followed by five or ten gentle breaths, while visualizing this inner muscle opening and relaxing. Next, continue through your remaining zones: your stomach muscles and diaphragm, your chest, your mouth and throat, and your eyes and forehead. Contract each group of muscles, and follow with five to ten gentle breaths. If you still feel stress after completing the five zones, continue in the reverse order, going through each zone again until you feel relaxed.

:60 Second Going Deeper Exercise: If you desire more emotional release, use the same techniques as in the previous example, but breathe with your mouth open. Each time you exhale, make a sighing sound that resonates in your throat to help release trapped feelings. Visualize your body in your mind, noting areas of tension, physical pain or deep-seated feelings. Treat all of these areas in the same fashion.

Try changing the sound of your sigh to reflect the different types of feelings in these areas. For example, let your sigh express the hurt and pain of a sore back, the anger at your boss trapped in your tight shoulders or the regret from having avoided speaking your mind. Continue to travel through these areas of your body, expressing the appropriate sound and sigh until you feel emotionally lighter and a slight tingling in your hands or feet. Once you have reached the state of light tingling, return to the belly-chest-exhale technique to help you relax and integrate your feelings.

FINDING YOUR INNER GROUND

The previous two :60 second breathing exercises are designed to promote relaxation and relieve emotional stress and old, trapped memories. The next step, following any release, is to transform this relaxation into increased self-confidence and inner strength.

While lying on your back, continue to breathe comfortably using the belly-chest-exhale technique. Visualize a miniature version of yourself, standing in the middle of your diaphragm. To find your diaphragm, find the point approximately two to three inches above your navel, just an inch or two below the inferior part of your breast bone. This is often called the *power center*, or the *spiritual center*, of the body in Buddhism and Hinduism. As you breathe, visualize your miniature self standing up, feeling strong and powerful. If any thoughts arise, let them go, and continue to focus on your miniature self standing on your inner ground.

If you want to proceed further, you might give a voice to this miniature self. Let your miniature self repeat a positive affirmation, such as, "I am strong, I am tall" or "With each breath, I become stronger and more secure." Obviously, the phrase is only important if it has meaning for you. Find a short phrase that expresses this strong self-speaking from your power center. When you have experienced the feeling of power, you will notice a deep breath rise up into your chest and a slight tingling in your arms or legs. At this point, you are finished and you may sit or stand. Take :60 seconds to really feel this inner strength before proceeding with your busy day-to-day activities and returning to your hectic lifestyle.

:60 SECOND BREATHING SUMMARY

- Heart and chest pain should always be taken very seriously; consult your physician if you experience these problems.
- In some cases, symptoms of a serious heart problem may actually signify a stress reaction.
- Breathing and heart rate are intimately related.
- Breathing is the primary function of your body which can be easily conscious or unconscious.
- Teach yourself how to breathe; teach yourself how to relax.
- Meditate when you feel stressed.
- Relax away stress using the :60 Second Rejuvenation Strategy's breathing techniques and five stress zone exercises.
- Achieve deeper emotional release using the same techniques and exercises—but add a deep audible sigh to help express deep-seated feelings.
- Find your inner self, give it a voice and stand on your inner ground.
- Memorize a positive affirmation—one that has meaning for you.

Chapter 4

STRETCHING FOR PAIN RELIEF—
:60 SECOND EXERCISES

:60 Second Affirmation:
"Stretching allows muscles to heal, emotions to surface."

Paul, a successful novelist, experienced occasional bouts of upper back and neck pain. A lucrative book contract from a New York publisher included stringent, monthly deadlines. Long, exhausting days wed to his computer were now regularly interrupted by vicious neck spasms. In desperation, he contacted me. He made it clear that he abhorred any type of regular exercise. I learned from talking to him that this was because he had only been taught old fashioned, mindless calisthenics and as a result had concluded that exercise had to be boring.

When I palpated Paul's middle back, upper back and neck, I came to the conclusion that much of his pain was due to the chronic muscle spasms in these areas. He needed a stretching program that would be simple, quick and easy to perform. I knew that loading him down with the burden of a strenuous series of exercises would promote rebellion. Paul was witty, brilliant and resistant, and he bored easily. I decided to prescribe only one exercise which required approximately ten seconds to perform. This one exercise involved stretching his upper back muscles, which were the center of his complaints. I showed him how to perform the ear-to-shoulder stretch to make certain that he felt the muscles in the painful area being elongated. Paul winced as he stretched his tight upper back muscles, acknowledging that it provoked his chronic pain.

After he finished performing this one stretch, I told him to return in two to three weeks to assess whether or not the stretch was of benefit. Paul looked at me incredulously and said, "Is that all you're going to give me?" I told him that I wanted him to develop a habit of stretching, not be overloaded with drudgery. I realized that Paul needed to learn that he had some control over his pain. By limiting his program to one exercise, I thought it would be more likely that he would see the cause and effect relationship between his muscle tension and his primary pain complaint.

Paul returned three weeks later to report that his upper back felt significantly improved. Now he complained of the pain in his neck and middle back, the regions above and below the area he had been stretching. Again, I only prescribed one exercise for each area. Paul asked that I give him at least two or three more, but I refused. I knew that if we continued by slowly increasing the vigor of his program, it would be more likely that he would understand how exercise could relieve his chronic, nagging backache and that he would continue to perform the exercises.

After four sessions, all of his pain was gone and I discharged him with a total of four stretching exercises which required a total of about :60 seconds to perform. Exercise is like all other disciplines. You will be likely to continue practicing any discipline if it is easy, quick to perform and yields results.

:60 SECOND EXERCISES

If you are performing the following six exercises consecutively you should be able to complete them in :60 seconds. All of the exercises are designed to stretch your entire spine quickly, easily and comfortably. None of the exercises should cause any pain, but they will result in improved posture and an increased sense of comfort and well-being. The following are the *basic six*.

The Pigeon

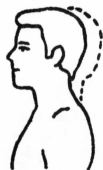

Tuck your chin slightly as you retract your head. If you find this difficult, try it lying down on your back. As your head retracts, you will feel pressure on the back of your skull. After you have pulled your head back for approximately one second, relax your neck muscles and allow your head to move forward. Performed correctly, the motion is similar to that of a walking pigeon.

Frequency: Perform three to five times per day.

Figure 4-1. The Pigeon

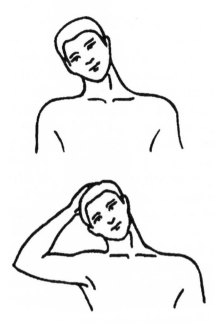

The Ear-to-Shoulder

Bend your neck to the right as if trying to place your right ear on your right shoulder. You will feel this stretch in the left side of your neck and upper back muscles. Hold for ten seconds and then try the stretch on the opposite side.

For a deeper stretch, place your right hand on top of your head, reaching over towards your left ear. Use your hand to very gently pull your head to to the right. Do not force the stretch or continue if you feel any pain or strain. Now, try the stretch on the opposite side.

Frequency: Perform three to five times per day.

Figure 4-2. The Ear-to-Shoulder

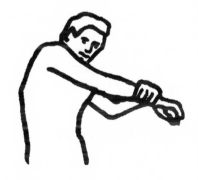

The Wrist Pull

With your arms extended straight out in front of you, grab your right wrist with your left hand. Gently round your back and pull your right wrist away from you. You should feel this stretch through your upper back and shoulders. Hold this stretch for ten to fifteen seconds before gently releasing. Now try this stretch on the opposite side.

Figure 4-3. The Wrist Pull

Frequency: Perform three to five times per day.

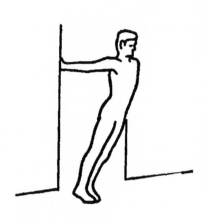

Figure 4-4. The Doorway Stretch

The Doorway Stretch

Elevate your right arm so that it is at a 90-degree angle to your body. Walk through a doorway, holding onto the doorframe with your right hand. Gently walk through the doorway, while continuing to hold onto the doorframe. Feel the stretch through your right chest muscles. For a deeper stretch, pull your body further from the doorway, leaning forward and on your toes, while still holding on with your right hand. If you feel any strain or pain, do not attempt to achieve this deeper stretch. Repeat the doorway stretch on your left side. This may also be performed on a wall, but you must turn your body slightly to the left to perceive a stretch.

Frequency: Perform three to five times per day.

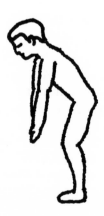

The Knee Touch

Stand with your feet hip-width apart. With your knees slightly bent, gently bend over while rounding your back, as if you are going to touch your knees. As you begin feeling a stretch through your back, stop moving and hold for a few seconds. Then, slowly return to the upright position.

Frequency: Perform for three to five times per day.

Figure 4-5. The Knee Touch

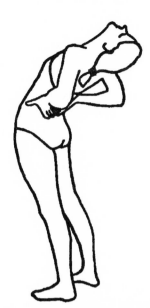

The Standing Back Bend

Stand with your feet hip-width apart. Place your hands on either side of your lower back, just above your pelvis. Gently lean back as you press forward on your lower back with your hands. Use your hands as a fulcrum to gently press each lumbar vertebra forward while you gently bend back. Once you feel a stretch through your back, hold for a moment before slowly returning to your original upright position.

Frequency: Perform for three to five times per day.

Figure 4-6. The Standing Back Bend

:60 SECOND NATURAL BENDING TECHNIQUE

The basic principles of bending, twisting, pushing and pulling involve learning to bend from your hips rather than from your back. Your hip sockets are powerful and well protected and do not possess the delicate disks and joints that exist in your lower back.

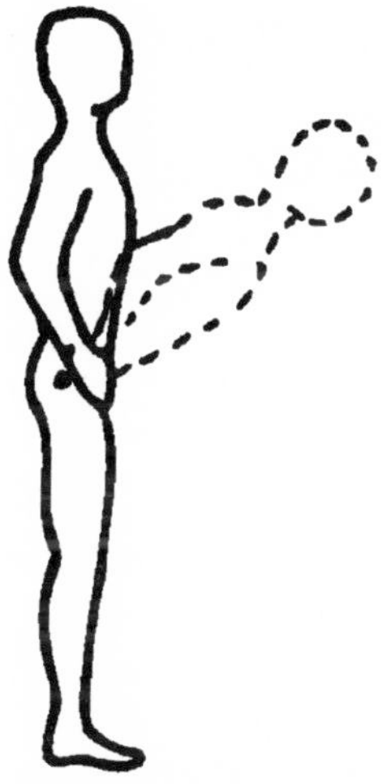

To practice this exercise, stand with your feet hip-width apart and your spine in neutral. With your knees slightly bent, find the large, bony protuberance on your hip, called the *greater trochanter*. To find it, draw a straight line down your side from your armpit to your bony pelvic brim. As you continue to move your hand down your pelvis, you will find a large bony bump approximately six inches below your pelvic brim.

Figure 4-7. Bending Forward, Rotating From an Imaginary Axis

Visualize that you are holding a pole in both of your hands that passes through your pelvis. This axis will be the center of your range of motion. Bend slightly forward, rotating from this imaginary axis. Be certain that you keep your spine in a neutral position throughout this bend by

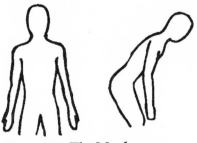

Figure 4-8. The Monkey

focusing your eyes along the wall in front of you and then to the floor in a smooth arc. When you have bent to an approximate 45-degree angle, hold then slowly straighten up, returning to the neutral standing position. This bending exercise should take approximately five to ten seconds.

Once this exercise becomes easy, drop your hands to your sides and repeat the motion. Some people like to visualize this forward bent position mimicking the posture of a monkey. After performing this exercise a few times, you are ready to try bending and twisting with your spine in neutral.

Notice in the diagram above how bending is accomplished in a comfortable, graceful manner without contorting or twisting the spinal column. This exercise should be performed a few times a day, :60 seconds per session until you feel comfortable bending with your spine in neutral.

The next time you need to empty the trunk of your car or grab something out of a low cabinet, try using this monkey exercise in addition to bending and lifting with your legs to prevent stress and strain.

:60 SECOND PAIN RELIEF SUMMARY

- Always stretch in a comfortable place using the belly-chest-exhale technique.
- When exhaling, sigh aloud or make a sound that reflects your feelings at the time.
- Allow emotions to surface, but do not force them; do not stifle a feeling when you sense it arising.
- Performing the *basic six*, three to five times per day, will keep you pain-free and productive.
- Performed consecutively, the *basic six* exercises should take :60 seconds to complete.
- Remember that you can often gain control over your pain and you have the power to heal yourself.
- Seek professional help if needed.
- Learn how to bend, twist, push and pull using proper posture.
- Learn to bend from your hips rather than from your back.
- Practice the monkey exercise for :60 seconds a few times a day.
- Remember the monkey exercise and try to incorporate it into daily activities that require bending, pushing or pulling.

PART 2

HARMONIZING MIND AND BODY

Chapter 5

THE MIND—CALM OR CHAOS?

:60 Second Affirmation:
"Calming my mind, my soul rejoices."

Nancy was a dedicated wife and mother. Although she adored her husband and two teenage boys, with the increasing challenges in her life, she began to go through periods of emotional stress and tension. These bouts of stress resulted in regular outbursts of anger, resulting in emotional distance from her family. Her husband expressed his bitterness and displeasure with her behavior and her sons began withdrawing from her, wanting to spend more time with their dad. Nancy was left feeling isolated at a time when she needed love and understanding.

Nancy described her problem, and I made the assumption that there was probably a depressive side to her anger. Depression is often anger turned inwards, while regular angry outbursts often arise from the depths of depression and desperation.

When I referred Nancy to a psychiatrist, she became upset. She described how she had been in psychotherapy for the last fifteen years, working diligently on all aspects of her behavior. However, I explained to her that the frequency of her outbursts was, more than likely, the result of a hormonal or biochemical imbalance, not psychological difficulty. In addition to sending her to a psychiatrist, I suggested techniques that gave Nancy alternative reactions to difficult situations.

One of the most helpful suggestions was to give her a wide variety of :60 second responses to any situation. I told her to first try accepting the situation. If that did not work, I encouraged her to leave the situation—to literally walk away from it. Then she could express her anger indirectly, either physically or verbally, without engaging in a confrontation with her family. If both of these processes failed, I encouraged her to go back and talk to her family and express her anger. I also encouraged her to try a number of other techniques for calming her mind. The remainder of this chapter discusses these mind-calming techniques.

MEDITATING WITHOUT MANTRAS

There has been an increasing interest in the practice of meditation. Medical doctors, psychologists and religious teachers extol its stress-reducing virtues. Yet meditation teachers often preach rigid, uncomfortable postures and arcane rituals. Most of us, when we think about meditation, still visualize burning incense and chanting mindless mantras. Or, we think of the torture of sitting cross-legged for hours in stony silence. This chapter will teach you how to enjoy the many benefits of meditation during your daily life activities. There is no need to engage in rigid, extended and uncomfortable practices to enjoy its benefits.

Meditating might seem like a difficult undertaking. But all you need are :60 second increments of time and a comfortable position. You may feel exhilarated following your first meditation session. You might feel peaceful and relaxed, or you might feel nothing whatsoever. Continue to practice this easy technique and you will, in a short time, be rewarded.

:60 Second Meditation Technique

Practice this :60 second technique while you are lying down in bed, upon awakening, as the beginning of an afternoon nap or before going to sleep in the evening. These techniques are so simple you can practice them while at work, while waiting in line at the bank, while exercising or even while sitting in your car. The reason meditation can fit into any aspect of your life is because you can meditate for as little as :60 seconds to begin or as long as sixty minutes if you have the time.

First, find the neutral position while standing, sitting or lying on your back. Once you have found this comfortable neutral position, close your eyes, take one very deep slow breath and then slowly exhale. This is the simplest act of meditation. That is why it can even be done in a traffic jam. As you know, when stuck in traffic, you may not move for minutes. Thus, taking a few seconds to find a comfortable neutral posture, closing your eyes and taking a relaxing breath can be a welcome interlude to the stress and drudgery of your commute. Obviously, do not close your eyes while traveling at high speeds on the expressway.

Because these techniques can be practiced in as little as five seconds, they can be practiced anywhere, any time. It will be more relaxing to give yourself at least :60 seconds to meditate, but even five seconds—such as a break from staring at your computer or a short interlude during a long wait on the telephone—can turn drudgery into pleasure. Let yourself feel that your daily, mundane tasks may be opportunities to relax and enjoy yourself.

Important :60 Second Points to Remember

1. Sit, stand or lie in the neutral position and close your eyes.
2. Be aware of the inhalation and exhalation of your breath.
3. Be aware of the pause between your inhalation and exhalation.
4. When thoughts arise, simply observe them and make no value judgments about them.
5. Continue to focus on the sensations in your body and mind as the breath moves in and out.
6. Open your eyes and feel refreshed.

More Advanced Suggestions

If you desire to pursue meditating for more than :60 seconds, here are a few suggestions:

> **Relieving Tension:** After finding the neutral sitting, standing or lying position, pay attention to your each of your five stress zones. Be certain that all of the muscles in these areas are relaxed.

> **Sitting:** The easiest way to sit is with proper support and posture in your car or your chair at work or at home. If you desire a more traditional approach, try sitting on a meditation cushion or bench. These are available in most cities at spiritually oriented bookstores. If you live in a small town, look on the internet under "meditation supplies."

> **Placement of Hands:** If you are sitting, place your hands in a comfortable position on your knees or in your lap. If you are standing

or lying down, place them in any position that you find comfortable. Whether your hands are interlocked or laying at your side is unimportant. Since meditation is a personal approach to relaxation and wellness, you must choose what feels comfortable for you.

Thinking: If you find thoughts interrupting your meditation, don't worry. Your mind is always thinking. However, if you continue to practice these techniques, you will eventually find that focusing on your breath will eventually allow those thoughts to simply drift away and become unimportant.

Distractions: If you have an itch, need to go to the bathroom or feel a need to move, don't worry. Scratch your itch, go to the bathroom or move until you find a comfortable position. Meditation does not require you to remain perfectly still to reap it's benefits.

Visualization: You might find that repeating a phrase, called a *mantra* helps you to relax. Words such as *peace, amen, om,* etc., are very popular. You might use one of these words or develop your own word or phrase like, "I am relaxing" or "I am letting go," to help you relax. It might also help to visualize an image which you find pleasing. Visualizing God, a rose or a beautiful scene are all appropriate and helpful if you find them soothing.

OTHER MIND-CALMING TECHNIQUES

Choosing a Teacher

Most religious practices, including Christianity, Judaism, Buddhism and Hinduism, all describe the benefits of working with a teacher. In Christianity and Judaism, that teacher would be your priest, minister or rabbi. People who regularly attend church have been found to recover faster from illness and suffer less psychological stress. In Eastern religions, the teacher, often called a guru, functions much like a minister, teaching how to find higher consciousness and educating about religious philosophy, as well as dealing with everyday life stresses and strains.

Spiritual Anchors

You will find that :60 second self-reminders about spiritual ideas can be quite helpful in keeping your mind focused on calming ideas. Place an *anchor* in every room to remind you to calm your mind. A crucifix on the wall, a picture of a guru, incense, candles, flowers, a beautiful sculpture or a tranquil painting can all be helpful. When you find stress overcoming you, redirect your attention to the calming influence of these important spiritual objects. Your consciousness of God or a higher plane of existence will put your day-to-day problems into perspective.

Confessions

There are three steps to confession: confess, feel remorse and resolve to avoid repeating the behavior (avoidance).

Confess

To confess, you must express, out loud or silently, what you have done wrong. It does not matter if the harmful behavior is small or large. It only matters that you feel some type of guilt, anguish or stress from the action. You might simply say, "I am sorry I hurt you" or "Forgive me for not being there for you," etc. It takes courage and humility to confess to a party you have wronged, but a confession can lead to resolution of negative feelings.

Feel Remorse

After you have confessed, it is important to feel your remorse. Remorse or guilt is like running a spiritual "temperature." Spend :60 seconds in silence and be aware of all of your bodily sensations. Pay attention to your five stress zones and your deepest feelings. You'll be more likely to finish this exercise with a very calm mind if you reflect on what you have done.

Resolve (Avoidance)

After you have felt the discomfort or psychological pain of your actions and are aware of how you have harmed another person, it is important to resolve to avoid that type of negative behavior in the future. Think about what caused you to engage in that worrisome or harmful activity and vow to avoid it in the future. Seek counseling or a support group such as Alcoholics Anonymous, a church, a stress management seminar, etc., to bolster your resolve and help you change.

Confessing your uncomfortable and harmful actions and resolving to avoid them in the future is only half of this mind-calming strategy. The other half is to forgive someone who you feel has hurt you in any way. It does not matter if you felt unloved as a child, suffered the rejection of a cherished lover or lost your job at the hands of an unfair boss. You will have difficulty being calm and happy unless you are free of anger and resentment and have forgiven the person who has harmed you.

Try telling one person that you felt hurt because of what he did, but you want him to know that you have no hard feelings and have forgiven him. Or, if this is difficult, repeat "I forgive you for what you have done" whenever a negative memory of that person or circumstance arises. Confessing and forgiving free the mind of guilt, anger and many other stressful emotions. Sometimes forgiving is hard work that takes some time, but the effort will be well worth it.

Don't Worry, Be Happy

Do something that you find fun. You will notice that after a pleasurable activity, your mind is clear and calm. It does not matter whether you go jogging, visit the local amusement park, watch a feel-good movie or go to a concert. Anything that you find fun will do. Often, in this hectic and stressful world, we become so focused on survival and work that we forget to do things that we find enjoyable.

Prayer

Whereas meditation involves clearing the mind, prayer involves filling the mind with requests to God or expressions of thankfulness. Because a prayer may only require a few seconds, it is a wonderful, efficient vehicle for calming your mind and getting in touch with higher powers. A long prayer helps you work through all the struggles of the heart and day and turn each one of them over to God's care. In this way you are no longer fighting your battles alone but have asked for God's help and power to guide and support you.

If you have never used prayer, merely close your eyes and take one or two breaths and say a :60 second incantation, "I pray that [you decide]." Praying for peace and harmony, a calm mind, a deeper connection with God or anything else you might desire can be quite helpful. Confession and forgiving can also be integrated into your prayer practice. Or you could make a :60 second list of all the things that are bothering you. Many people find reading the Bible combined with prayer totally quiets the mind and leads to inner peace and confidence.

Anger vs. Acceptance

One of the reasons that religion and spiritual practice can be helpful for calming the mind occurs because of its emphasis on acceptance. Assuming that a situation is due to God's will or caused by a power greater than yourself can relieve you of feeling responsible for everything. When a situation arises that is disturbing, you have a choice of reacting or accepting the situation, knowing that even if it is unpleasant at the time, you may learn something valuable from it.

To accept the situation, resist saying or doing anything. If you have trouble accepting the situation, try saying to yourself, "I accept this situation" or something similar. Later, when you have time, meditate around that situation or pray as often as necessary until one day you find you are at peace with it.

Sometimes it is impossible to accept a situation. Often, an unacceptable situation will cause anger or resentment. This anger or resentment needs to be expressed in non-destructive ways when you feel the pressure building inside of you. Like a bottle of soda that is shaken vigorously, this pressure, if not relieved, will burst out often in a destructive manner. There are non-destructive ways to deal with anger. You can relieve this pressure either directly or indirectly.

Direct anger involves telling someone why you are angry with them, but only after you have given yourself a chance to calm down. This is the most direct way to express your anger and often provides the most rapid resolution. However, expressing a tremendous amount of anger to your boss or to your child may be counterproductive. If you feel this type of anger is inappropriate, try the indirect approach.

Indirect anger involves expressing your feelings when you are alone. You might try writing about your feelings, closing the windows of your car and screaming, vigorously exercising, pounding a pillow on your bed or imagining you are talking to a person while in the quiet privacy of your own home. Sometimes this method is very useful for getting your angry emotions out and then you are better able to approach the person you are angry with in order to achieve a resolution. Attempt a peaceful resolution whenever you can. Remember, most anger is caused by miscommunication or misunderstanding, so be prepared to think the best of people and to listen to and appreciate their point of view—not just your own.

:60 SECOND CALMING SUMMARY

- Either accept a situation, leave the situation or express your anger regarding the situation.
- Expressing anger can be effectively accomplished either directly or indirectly.
- Learn how to forgive and forget.
- Calm your mind with prayer, enjoyable activities, spiritual anchors and releasing of anger.
- The three steps to confession are: confess, feel remorse and resolve to avoid the detrimental act or behavior (avoidance).
- Learn how to breathe.
- Learn how to quiet your mind.
- Learn to meditate.
- Learn the true meaning of relaxation.
- Turn daily mundane tasks into opportunities to relax and enjoy yourself.

Chapter 6

DECISION MAKING—
AVOIDING AMBIVALENCE AND PAIN

:60 Second Affirmation:
"My mind is blind; my heart knows."

Bill had finally achieved a modicum of success. He had passed the difficult examination required to manage and sell real estate. However, he shared with me that he was having second thoughts about his impending marriage to his fianceé, Cheryl. Throughout their three years of courtship, there had been continual fights and bickering over life decisions–nothing was easy. Now, with two weeks to go before his wedding, he was getting cold feet. His relatives on both sides were planning to fly in from many parts of the United States for this joyous occasion. An added complication concerned his devout Christian faith and his African-American heritage. He felt that breaking off the wedding was similar to divorce, a behavior he obviously rejected.

He was surrounded by friends and relatives that had suffered the pain of divorce, which added to his fear. Because he had never known his own father, he was determined to be a loving father and faithful husband. Yet he could not seem to shake his insecurity about his rapidly approaching wedding day. I explained to Bill how to make this decision in less than :60 seconds, using what I call the Yes/No Rule.

THE :60 SECOND YES/NO RULE

The basic principle of the *Yes/No Rule* is that decisions should not be based upon ambivalent emotions. It is far better to take no action than take the wrong action. Even if we proceed through life with certainty of spirit and purpose, we will still meet challenges and doubts along the path. However, ambivalence is usually a sign that we anticipate that problems will occur. I explained this to Bill and told him to use the Yes/No Rule with the following principles:

> Yes = Yes
> No = No
> Uncertainty = No

If you are convinced that the decision is right, then the answer is "yes." It is impossible to know whether or not you made the correct decision, but with the certainty that you have made the right choice you will be likely to experience a positive outcome. If your answer to a decision or question is absolutely "no" then you can also feel comfortable with your decision. The problem comes when there is ambivalence. If you vacillate between yes and no, feel indecisive or can't make up your mind, take no action—the answer is "no."

Use the Yes/No Rule whenever you feel in a quandary about a decision. Remember that yes means yes, no means no, and ambivalence always means no. There is a legend that says that Buddha once remarked, "Don't just do something, stand there."

The Yes/No Rule is a helpful paradigm when you need to make a decision that is binary. A binary decision is one which only has two possible responses—yes or no. Ambivalence is a holding pattern prior to making one of those two choices. Sometimes ambivalence is an inner voice signal that says you haven't made up your mind yet. In that case, accept the fact that you have not decided yet what to do. Give yourself time to make a decision. If your feelings remain ambivalent, the answer is "no."

THE :60 SECOND ICE CREAM RULE

Unlike the Yes/No Rule, which is designed to help you make a decision with only two choices, the *Ice Cream Rule* is designed to help you choose when there are many possible responses. The basic principle of the Ice Cream Rule is that making a choice among a host of possibilities is really as easy as choosing between chocolate, vanilla and strawberry ice cream. When choices are many, you need to learn to recognize what sensation inside of you is associated with desire.

To master the Ice Cream Rule, first start with something simple. Next time you are asked an easy question, notice how you proceed in finding the answer. Take something simple, such as your choice of ice cream, political party or your favorite drink. You will probably find the answer in one of your five stress zones. For example:

> If you are asked whether 2 plus 2 equals 1, 2, 3 or 4, you will answer this question using your first stress zone. You will think about it, thus your brain is the source of energy or sensation for that decision.

> Any time you taste a food or drink, your tastebuds, your mouth and your nose have recorded the flavor, smell and sensation. In fact, tasty food will make you salivate, another sign that your second stress zone is active. You use your mouth and nose to make these types of decisions.

> When you observe something inspiring, a mother with her young baby or a heroic act, you will feel your heart react with love, warmth or pride. Those sensations stir in your third stress zone.

> The stomach and the intestines make up your fourth stress zone. It is the center of fear and anxiety, as well as sensuality and openness. Your fourth stress zone will tighten when you are fearful or anxious and it will relax when you are happy and open.

> Your fifth stress zone is your center of survival and sexuality. What happens when you become physically attracted to someone? Most people report some type of arousal, such as tingling, pulsating or some other type of physiological response. You will find that your fifth stress zone will tell you about your attraction to that person.

Your five stress zones can help you make choices in life. By paying attention to your bodily sensations and understanding what sensation signifies attraction and what sensation signifies avoidance, you will be able to resolve indecision.

You will sense whether you are in a state of attraction or avoidance. If you start seeing each choice as being something you are attracted to or something you prefer to avoid, and then pair it with a bodily sensation, you will find decision making much easier and more pleasurable. It will become as easy as choosing between chocolate, vanilla and strawberry ice cream.

THE :60 SECOND DEATH RULE

The Yes/No Rule may be inappropriate for more complex decisions. And these decisions may not fit into the Ice Cream Rule, which helps you choose any number of possibilities. If all else fails, try the :60 Second Death Rule.

The Death Rule is based upon the basic principle that most people, as they approach death, feel content about some aspects of their life and also feel remorse about other things. This is a natural human tendency—to look back on your life and evaluate your actions, with death as your judge and jury.

But why wait for the moment before death to use this wisdom? You can use a visualization to help you attain some of the same enlightenment. Lie on your back in your bed or some other quiet place and visualize yourself lying on your death bed. What do you think you would say if you were to look back from your death bed to the here and now? How would you view your problems, your decisions and your choices? The Death Rule is a simple principle. It teaches you that you can use the wisdom of death to make your life more meaningful and worthwhile. While it sounds a bit morbid, the Death Rule will actually help you live more richly, kindly and morally.

:60 SECOND DECISION-MAKING SUMMARY

- Use the Yes/No Rule, the Ice Cream Rule or the Death Rule to make a decision.
- Remember that Yes = Yes, No = No, and Uncertainty = No.
- Ambivalence is usually a sign that we anticipate problems will occur or that we have not given ourselves time enough to reach a conclusion.
- You will probably find the answer to your dilemma in one of your stress zones.
- Use the death rule to resolve more complex problems or those that cannot be resolved using the Yes/No Rule or the Ice Cream Rule.

Chapter 7

DIETING—THE EASY WAY

:60 Second Affirmation:
"Focusing on a primitive diet, I grow strong."

Jim had moved to California from Atlanta, Georgia to teach at Stanford University. At Stanford, he developed a sterling reputation as an exciting professor of Cultural Anthropology. Students invariably rated him as the most interesting teacher at the university. Jim's specialty was South American Indians, especially rituals and witchcraft. But Jim's brilliance was confined to his stunning intellectual capacity. He confided in me that he was emotionally insecure, although he disguised it well with his wit and intellectual insight.

Jim was quite overweight and mentioned that he wanted to lose weight as I worked on his stiff neck. I discussed various types of weight-loss regimens with Jim—the high protein diet, the vegetarian diet, the Zone diet and many of the other available regimens. But Jim was an iconoclast; he was rebellious. He said he had difficulty following any diet that seemed as strict as a religious practice. So I began to explain to Jim the basic evolution of human nutrition and how our modern diet has evolved. Jim's interest in anthropology was stimulated by this discussion. He thanked me for our enlightening discussion and for fixing his neck and rushed off to teach his class at the university.

Jim returned approximately five months later with lower back pain. When he walked in my office, I was quite surprised. He had lost about thirty *pounds and appeared drastically more fit and trim. When I inquired about his appearance, he told me that the regimen we discussed had changed his attitude toward food. I did not realize that I had given him a diet. But, as I thought about it hours later, I realized primitive man had evolved to a very natural dietary regimen that could be learned and followed quite easily. As Jim said to me, "I can teach someone this diet in :60 seconds or less."*

THE DIETARY DILEMMA

We are bombarded with thousands of diets. Each diet has a philosophy of eating with a physiological explanation. However, this explanation is often in conflict with other competing diet strategies. Rather than trying to follow each new diet, it makes more sense to study our primitive ancestors, how we have evolved and how our diet has changed. The diet in the *:60 Second Rejuvenation Strategy* is based upon eating foods that anthropological research has shown are most compatible with human life.

THE HISTORY OF DIET

An article on Paleolithic Nutrition in the *New England Journal of Medicine* noted that many of the major diseases of modern society, such as heart problems, high blood pressure, obesity and cancer may be based upon faulty nutrition. They concluded that there is an inextricable relationship between evolution and the human diet. There have been very few changes in our genetic makeup in the last 100,000 years. However, there has been a dramatic change in our diet. The modern-day diet may be incompatible with our biological make up, thus increasing the incidence of many serious diseases.

Clara Davis studied the self-selected diets of young children and found that they would naturally choose a healthy, nutritionally balanced diet when they were provided choices of various nutritious and unprocessed foods. When they were presented with very sweetened, less natural foods, they had difficulty eating in a balanced fashion. Young children, and probably many adults as well, have the ability to survive on a wide variety of foods. Yet choosing to eat the healthier foods may not be easy—especially when most of us grow up eating foods loaded with fat and sugar.

THE PRIMITIVE SOLUTION

Millions of years ago, primitive man would wander and forage for food. He had not learned how to use fire for cooking and had no concept of the idea of cultivating food. His diet consisted of wild fruits, uncooked vegetables and raw meats. These were the only foods available. Living like most animals, the majority of his day was spent searching for food.

Archeological evidence clearly describes early humans as being omnivores, eating both animal and plant products. Fossils of early humans, from as much as 2,000,000 years ago indicate a species biased toward eating both small animals and plant foods. Later, stone tools were used to butcher and prepare the carcasses of larger animals. Meat was then eaten with wild fruits and vegetables that could be foraged from nearby plants. This is similar to the diet of most humans today, although we have found easier ways to obtain food and prepare it.

Anthropologists agree that early humans relied on plants for the bulk of their subsistence, supplementing this with meats whenever possible. The tremendous amount of protein, vitamins and minerals present in meat made it an ideal nutritional source to develop strength and endurance—important factors for primitive man. Plants provided additional, complex nutrients called *phytochemicals*, as well as vitamins, minerals and roughage.

Many researchers now believe *Homo sapiens* appeared approximately 50,000 years ago. Because they were nearly identical to human beings of today, it is relevant to understand their eating habits. Our *Homo sapien* ancestors, like ourselves, were able to perceive the four basic tastes of sweet, salt, sour and bitter.

Being able to distinguish between these tastes was an important factor in human evolution. Many bitter plants are poisonous, while sweet, tasty fruits and vegetables are generally fresh, edible and nutritious. By contrast, spoiled food has a bitter or sour taste which is very unpleasant. Our ancestors learned, through trial and error (or death), to appreciate foods that were nutritious and avoid unhealthy, potentially dangerous, toxic or poisonous foods. Early man must have spent much of his time foraging, sampling and only then choosing that which tasted pleasant.

EVOLUTION AND MALNUTRITION

Unlike humans today, our primitive ancestors, the *Homo sapiens*, were required to spend most of their day engaged in vigorous physical exercise scrounging for their food. After this vigorous workout, and if they were lucky enough to find a bounty of food, they would feast on wild vegetables, fruits and lean meats. Thus, if a variety of food was abundant, not only was their diet healthy, the manner in which they had to obtain it contributed to their strength and fitness.

However, many thousands of years later, man developed farms. Cohen and Arnelagos, in their study of the "Origins of Agriculture," concluded that early farmers often suffered nutritional deficiencies and osteoporosis. By developing a more limited range of foods, especially an increased consumption of grains, they began to deviate from the natural diet. This relatively recent transition into the science of food production has created a diet which is overly processed and unnatural.

Today we are bombarded by processed and engineered foods, loaded with calories and artificial flavors, to tempt our desire for salt, fat and sugar. These tastes are craved by most people, because our primitive instincts believe that they contain less toxicity. However, the irony is that these engineered foods contain preservatives and chemicals which may have harmful side effects.

THE IDEAL DIET—THE PRIMITIVE SOLUTION

If we focus on the science of nutritional evolution, we can learn how to eat healthy food, lose weight, feel better and live a long and healthy life. By observing a few, simple rules, requiring :60 seconds to learn, you can improve your health and avoid plodding through hundreds of diet books.

Focus on Fruits and Vegetables

Modern research has documented that fruits and vegetables contain compounds called *phytochemicals*. These compounds are like vitamins and minerals, but can only be found in fruits and vegetables. These foods have been documented to lower the risk of heart disease, and help prevent nearly all types of cancers. Fruits and vegetables contain phytochemicals, vitamins and minerals in abundance. Therefore, they should be the primary focus of your diet. If you feel like a snack, you can stuff yourself full of carrots and celery without worry. Fruits and vegetables should be eaten with every meal and in large quantities. This should be the primary focus of your diet. If possible, choose organic fruits and vegetables free of pesticides and other toxic sprays.

Supplement with Lean Meat

It is difficult to get sufficient Vitamin C in your diet without eating fresh fruits and vegetables. It is also very difficult to get Vitamin B_{12} without eating meat products. Even heart doctors recommend eating small amounts of lean meat on a regular basis for this reason. They counsel their patients with heart disease and high blood pressure to avoid fatty meats, and eat more poultry and lean fish. If you can find meats free of hormones and other toxic chemicals, that is ideal. Most major grocery chains and health food stores carry meats and poultry free of hormones and medication.

Egg phobia

Eggs can also be safely included in a healthy diet. An egg only has five grams of fat and is a great food for promoting weight loss if eaten in moderation. Just make sure that you fry or scramble your eggs without butter (or better yet, poach or boil them) and you will provide yourself with a valuable source of nutrition—six grams of protein and valuable vitamins and minerals. Many years ago, doctors thought eggs were bad for the heart. Now we know the truth. People who eat eggs regularly have cholesterol no higher than those who avoid eggs for low-calorie dishes. Compare a scrambled egg to a typical dessert. Want a slice of cheesecake? That's almost fifteen grams of fat. How about a candy bar? That will cost you about ten to fifteen grams of fat. Just remember to eat eggs only in modest amounts and as a supplement to your primary diet, which should be fruits, vegetables and whole grains. You can have an egg a couple of times per week and not feel guilty.

Everything Else

Eat small amounts of everything else. Pasta, bread, cheese and other processed foods should be eaten sparingly. This does not mean you cannot have a glass of wine and enjoy cheese and crackers! Even primitive man inadvertently ate toxic foods when he was surprised by a poisonous plant or unknowingly ate spoiled or diseased meat. You have the ability to eat almost anything because your body is so able to adapt to a wide variety of foodstuffs. Just don't allow these other foods to become your sole source of nutrition. Remember, your primary diet should be vegetables, fruits and lean meats.

PRIMITIVE BREAKFAST

Fruit is a beneficial way to start your day. Although the medical research on their health risks and benefits are continually changing, eggs, with their powerful protein and vitamin content, are also an excellent breakfast food if cholesterol permits. Intersperse fruit and eggs with occasional lean meats, such as turkey sausage, and whole grains. Oatmeal and other popular cereals can be eaten occasionally.

LUNCH

If a hectic schedule occasionally forces you to eat fast food, get a salad with your sandwich and either use whole wheat bread or remove at least one of the slices. Remember to supplement even your fast food with lots of fruits and vegetables. Snacking on an apple, banana or another type of fruit after lunch is a very healthy addition to your sandwich. Because soups often contain small amounts of meats with lots of vegetables, they also should be considered an important part of a diet which seeks to imitate a primitive one.

DINNER

Because meat, poultry or fish is a typical evening meal in most parts of the world, it is easy for dinner to be a primitive meal. However, it is wise to move away from serving and eating red meat, like steak and hamburger, and increase the frequency of poultry and fish at your dinner table. With your portion of lean meat, eat copious amounts of cooked vegetables or salad and snack on some fresh fruit for dessert.

FOODS TO AVOID

One of my first teachers was an osteopathic physician who had one motto when asked about nutrition. He would quickly retort, "If it don't rot, don't eat it." This simple statement was truly filled with wisdom. Try to avoid all foods that don't spoil. All of the foods eaten by our ancestors would have rotted when exposed to the open, warm air. Try to avoid canned and packaged foods, except on rare occasions. Avoid highly processed foods and foods with preservatives or artificial flavor or coloring.

INDIVIDUAL VARIATION

You are a unique individual and no one possesses your exact genetic structure. Therefore, you must experiment with different types of foods to assess which of the primitive foods you find most pleasant and tasty. Each of your five stress zones can help you understand which of these primitive foods is right for you.

Zone 1

Your brain is part of Zone 1. Think about the foods that you eat. Remember to follow the primitive diet, eating lots of fruits and vegetables, supplemented by lean meats and eggs. Occasionally sample all types of foods for variety.

Zone 2

Smell and taste are an important part of this stress zone. Realize that your genetic makeup will make you favor sweet and salty foods, so attempt to resist your unhealthy temptations. Try to eat fruits and vegetables, and meat or eggs rather than sweet and salty snack foods. Try to create a relaxing atmosphere and focus on enjoying your meal. Taste things very carefully and try not to engage in other activities while eating. Take time to chew slowly. This will give your second stress zone a chance to more accurately taste food and fully enjoy it without distraction.

Zone 3

It is not uncommon for people who have allergies to eat certain foods that can cause wheezing, coughing or other symptoms in the third stress zone. Eating large portions of wheat or dairy products, certain types of nuts or seeds, shellfish and some fruits may cause this reaction. It may take twenty-four hours for your chest to react to an allergic food. If you have allergies, pay closer attention to the types of foods you eat to see if they have any correlation with your symptoms and consult a physician.

Zone 4

Primitive man worried about poisonous plants, probably ate a tiny bit of a new food and waited a few minutes to assess the reaction of his stomach. Vomiting is a violent reaction to a toxic food. However, milder types of stomach upsets such as gurgling, gas and discomfort, can all be signs of a reaction in the fourth stress zone.

Zone 5

Constipation and diarrhea can happen fairly quickly or take up to two or three days to occur. It is common for too much coffee or spicy foods to cause diarrhea, while eating large amounts of bread, pasta, nuts and meats can cause constipation. The simplest antidote for constipation is to eat more fruits and vegetables, the most important part of the primitive diet.

:60 SECOND PRIMITIVE DIET SUMMARY

- The four basic tastes are sweet, salt, sour and bitter.
- We prefer the taste of sweet fruits and vegetables as did primitive man because it meant that the item was fresh and edible.
- Eat fruits and vegetables in abundance at every meal.
- Supplement meals regularly with lean meat, fish, poultry and eggs.
- All processed foods including pasta, bread and cheese should be eaten sparingly.
- Avoid canned or packaged foods, highly processed foods and foods that contain preservatives or artificial flavors or colorings.
- Fill up on fresh fruits and vegetables, lose weight and prevent heart attacks and cancer—all at the same time.
- Try baking, broiling or poaching instead of frying meats, poultry, fish and eggs.
- Beans, tofu, whole grains, nuts and seeds are all great sources of nutrition.
- If you think you have a food allergy but cannot identify the problem food, consult a physician or allergist for testing.

Chapter 8

EAT CAREFULLY
AND THOUGHTFULLY—
FOOD CAN ALTER YOUR MOOD

:60 Second Affirmation:
"I don't eat health food, I eat healthy food."

Lenore was an avid runner and cyclist. Every year she was a top finisher in Hawaii's Iron Man Triathlon. A seasoned and well-trained athlete, she spent many hours a day strengthening and stretching her powerful body. But then she began complaining of fatigue. She was losing interest in running and lacking the motivation to do anything.

I asked her to describe her typical breakfast, lunch and dinner. Like many athletes, she was preoccupied with carbohydrate loading, the practice of eating far more carbohydrates such as pasta, rice and bread than protein or fat. She told me that carbohydrate loading gave her instant energy and improved her mood. However, I suspected that her diet was out of balance. As I explained to her about the :60 Second Rejuvenation Strategy, I told her to focus on a more natural, less processed diet emphasizing fruits and vegetables, supplementing her diet with lean meat, chicken or turkey and fish. I explained to her that even eggs, nuts and seeds, in small amounts, could be extremely helpful. She initially resisted my suggestion. After all, she had been taught that carbohydrates could provide long, sustained energy.

Two weeks later, she returned to my office—ecstatic over the change. Her energy had returned, she felt leaner and less bloated and was again lifting *weights and jogging regularly. She added that although pasta and bread gave her a quick burst of energy, she felt her new eating habits gave her far more long-term endurance and consisted of foods that were easier to digest.*

THE FIVE/FIFTY FORMULA

The American Cancer Society suggests that you have five servings of fruits and vegetables daily. If you have a piece of fruit for breakfast, a carrot with lunch, a piece of fruit for a late afternoon snack and a salad or two vegetables with dinner, you have eaten your five servings. Think of a serving as the size of an average piece of fruit. Being precise is not as important as eating a wide variety of fruits and vegetables, even if the servings are small. I call this the Five/Fifty Formula because approximately fifty percent of your diet should be fruits and vegetables (five servings per day), including whole grains such as oats and rice. Processed grains do not count. Pasta, white bread and other processed foods have lost much of their nutrition during processing. Thus your diet should be composed of the following elements:

1. Large amounts of fruits, vegetables, brown rice, oatmeal and other whole grains. In fact, if you are trying to lose weight, eat as much of these foods as you desire. These are all very low in calories and high in fiber, and will promote vigorous health while you lose weight.
2. Moderate amounts of lean meats, fish and poultry, eggs, seeds and nuts.
3. Occasional indulgence in pasta, dairy products, breads and other fast foods and fatty foods.

The *:60 Second Rejuvenation Strategy* does not preach total elimination of pasta, processed foods, dairy products, breads, fast foods and fatty foods from your diet. It encourages you, however, to primarily eat fruits, vegetables and lean meats.

Food Allergies

If testing your five stress zones does not give you enough information about problem foods which are causing a mild negative reaction, you may need to do further testing. Try avoiding the suspicious food for at least two days. Then eat that food again, noting any reaction during the following twenty-four hours. Once you've pinpointed the problem food, eliminate it from your diet. If you have trouble finding the cause of your problem or if you are having a strong allergic reaction to something, consult a medical doctor or an allergist for testing.

Why This System Will Work

This diet is easy to follow. There is no need for a calculator, no reason to purchase a scale, and no calories to count. Fruits and vegetables are loaded with vitamins, minerals, trace elements and phytochemicals. These nutrients are packed with life-giving vitality, yet they have almost no fat or calories.

For example, a carrot has almost one gram of protein, but only a tenth of a gram of fat. Ten carrots will only provide one gram of fat. Compare this to a half cup of ice cream which may contain fifteen to twenty-five grams of fat. You would need to eat 250 carrots to equal one half cup of ice cream.

One stalk of celery also has approximately one-tenth of a gram of fat. Hungry? Feel like stuffing yourself? Get a whole head of lettuce, throw in a few slices of tomato, grate a carrot or two and drench it in non-fat salad dressing. You can get creative and add sliced fresh fruit, fresh mushrooms, chopped green or red onion, sliced radish or maybe even some sesame seeds, sunflower seeds or nuts. You can fill up on these foods and still only be eating one or two grams of fat. This large salad, big enough to feed a hungry family of four, has less than one-tenth the fat of a half cup of ice cream—but is loaded with nutrition.

If you are like most people, you have a sweet tooth. To the many people who are brought up eating sugared cereal, sweetened drinks and rich desserts, and find it difficult to eat enough vegetables, I would suggest starting with fruit. A fresh apple has approximately one-quarter to one-half gram of fat but is loaded with fiber, vitamins and minerals. There is a good reason for the old saying, "An apple a day keeps the doctor away."

How about strawberries? A half cup of strawberries has one-third gram of fat, one hundred times less fat than a half cup of ice cream. Next time you are in the supermarket, splurge on a basket of fresh strawberries. For a delicious dessert, buy some fruit-flavored non-fat yogurt and use it in place of whipped cream as a tasty topping. Add a ripe banana to this and you add only a half a gram of fat. Filling up on fresh fruits and vegetables will help you lose weight, prevent heart attacks and decrease your risk of getting cancer—all at the same time!

Proteins

Although the majority of your diet should be fruits and vegetables, lean meats also have an important place in your diet. In fact, an article published in the *International Journal of Vitamin and Nutritional Research* concluded that delaying the inclusion of meat in the diet of children after eight months of age seemed to be associated with iron deficiency when these children entered preschool. Although I am not advocating giving children large quantities of meat, small amounts of meat are an extremely valuable source of nutrition.

A study published in the *British Journal of Nutrition* in 1998 noted that mothers who regularly ate fish had a lower incidence of children born with a specific type of birth defect. They concluded that lean meats and cereals may help the fetal brain develop properly.

Adding lean meats and poultry to your diet will provide valuable vitamins and minerals, gobs of protein, tons of calcium and very little fat. A boneless roasted chicken breast without the skin has approximately one gram of fat. Compare this to a piece of fried chicken, which can easily have ten to twenty grams of fat. As you can see, eating poultry or meat is not the problem—it simply depends upon your method of preparation. Try to always purchase lean chicken or turkey. If you grill the meat and remove the skin and fat, you have a delicious source of valuable nutrients which is very low in fat. It is the perfect food for your diet.

Fish is also an extremely valuable source of nutrients and can prevent heart disease and cancer. A salmon burger has approximately one-half gram of fat. A mouth-watering salmon steak which has been baked, broiled or poached, only has five to ten grams of fat. Even though salmon has more fat than chicken or turkey, it has been shown to contain valuable oils that help prevent heart disease and cancer. Tuna is an especially low-fat fish. A quarter cup of canned tuna which has been packed in water has approximately one-half gram of fat. Atlantic and Pacific halibut only have two to three grams of fat per serving. As you can see, lean meats such as fish, chicken and turkey are a valuable source of nutrition, are low in fat and can help you lose weight.

Beans are another tremendous source of protein. Whether you eat bean soup, bean dip or baked beans, you will find them to be very satisfying and very low in fat. Another fantastic source of protein which is loaded with vitamins and minerals is tofu. Although many people think it tastes somewhat bland, try experimenting with tofu or soy protein in your favorite recipes. Sautéed with soy sauce or a Chinese marinade can produce a delicious main course. Soy products have been documented to reduce the risk of all types of cancers and lower cholesterol.

CHANGING THE WAY YOU SHOP

The easiest way to follow the :60 *Second Rejuvenation Strategy* diet is to steer your shopping cart straight for the fruit and vegetable section when you enter the supermarket. Load up your cart with luscious fresh fruits and vegetables first. Then wheel your cart swiftly over to the meat and fish section. If you have any questions, ask the butcher or meat clerk for the leanest cuts possible. Supplement these wholesome small portions of meat, fish and poultry products with a small amount of nuts and seeds.

Rice and oats should be considered whole grains and can be eaten regularly. Brown rice is better than white rice and slow-cooking oats are better than instant. However, if time is short, buy instant oats and instant rice. They are far better than any fast food and still contain valuable nutrients. Then as you wheel your cart away from the grains and cereals, try to avoid the processed pastas and sugar-laden cereals.

Feel free to buy eggs and low-fat or non-fat dairy products. Although your primary foods should consist of fruits, vegetables, lean meats, poultry, fish and grains, dairy products also provide an excellent source of calcium and can be low in fat. Many people are allergic to dairy products and react with gas, bloating or phlegm. For this group, you can either avoid eating dairy products altogether or consult your doctor about taking one of the newer medications that may help you better tolerate dairy products.

The Substitution Strategy

Another strategy for losing weight is to substitute more natural, lower-fat products for similar foods with less nutritional value. For example:
1. Substitute lean chicken, turkey or fish for beef and pork. You can even buy ground chicken or turkey to make your own low fat "hamburgers" or meatloaf or purchase ready-made turkey sausage or salmon burgers.
2. Try experimenting with vegetarian meat substitutes like vegetable protein or tofu. These low-fat, high-protein products can be substituted for meat in your favorite recipe.
3. Substitute fruit for fatty or sugary desserts. Rather than having one cup of ice cream, choose a half-cup of sorbet, frozen yogurt or low-fat ice cream with a half-cup of fresh fruit.
4. Choose low-fat or non-fat dairy products. They contain similar amounts of nutrients and protein as their higher fat counterparts, but are less likely to result in weight gain. Even if

you dislike the taste or consistency of skim or low-fat milk, there is no reason to drink fattening milk; there are milk products that offer the rich, thick taste of whole milk with the same low-fat content of 1% or skim milk.

5. Snack on fresh fruits and vegetables. All fruits and many vegetables such as celery and carrots are delicious, crunchy snack foods. Consider making a non-fat vegetable dip or even using a fruit-flavored yogurt as a dip for your vegetables.

6. Substitute slow cooking oatmeal, if you have the time, or instant oatmeal for sugary cereal.

7. Eat your largest meals for breakfast and lunch and eat a light dinner.

8. Substitute beans or legumes for meat.

Junk Food

The :60 *Second Rejuvenation Strategy* does not espouse completely avoiding ice cream, candy, cookies and other tempting sweets. Nor does it advise against having a steak once in awhile. Just make sure that your primary diet, using the Five/Fifty Formula, consists of fresh fruits and vegetables, supplemented by modest amounts of lean meats, poultry, and fish, eggs, seeds and nuts. Occasionally add rice, oats and low fat dairy products to your diet.

With the :60 *Second Rejuvenation Strategy*, nutritious eating becomes a lifestyle rather than a short, painful dieting experience which is prone to failure.

DIET AND DEPRESSION

At the Center for Human Nutrition in England, men and women alternated low-fat and moderate-fat diets every other month. The results suggested that low-fat diets created increased anger and hostility. A similar result was noted at the Bowman Gray School of Medicine in North Carolina, where researchers concluded that low cholesterol levels are associated with increased suicide and accidents. They speculated that very low cholesterol induce a mechanism designed to increase hunting or foraging behavior in the face of nutritional threat. A decline in cholesterol was viewed by the body as a threat, requiring aggressive action. They came to two startling implications for public health:

1. Low cholesterol could pose a risk of suicide or traumatic death.
2. Cholesterol lowering could result in impulsive or violent behavior.

An article in the *International Journal of Eating Disorders* had a very pertinent solution to this problem. They felt that some individuals could obtain a more permanent control of negative mood states by eliminating simple carbohydrates from their diet. These studies point out the truth in the *:60 Second Rejuvenation Strategy*—a diet emphasizing processed foods, lacking sufficient protein and fat, is unhealthy. A healthy diet should be supplemented by natural proteins and fats.

The Sugar Blues

Many people are quite sensitive to the effects of sugar. If you love sweet foods or crave desserts, you are part of this sugar-loving group. Remember that foods made with white flour, many cereals and most breads are very simple carbohydrates that increase your blood sugar level. Even that regular glass of wine or cola may be masking your sugar sensitivity.

Sugar-craving individuals may often feel depressed, sad or lethargic. Yet depression and lethargy are commonly treated with anti-depressant medication, not proper nutrition. These medications seek to balance your serotonin level. Serotonin is a brain chemical that, when secreted, creates a feeling of relaxation and inner peace. When serotonin levels are low, it is common to feel depressed, impulsive and edgy. Prozac, Serzone, Zoloft and Paxil are all popular antidepressants which modify the serotonin level in your brain.

If you are taking one of these serotonin-modifying drugs and are eating a high carbohydrate diet which is low in fat and protein, you might consider adding more protein to your diet. The *:60 Second Rejuvenation Strategy* diet will encourage you to avoid processed carbohydrates and focus instead on fruits and vegetables with lean meats. This will help stabilize your blood sugar level.

Pasta and Pain

If you cannot break the cycle of carbohydrate and sugar dependence, you will continue to feel weak, moody and lethargic. Because your metabolism has been distorted by improper diet, you will not achieve relief by taking medication or pumping up your blood sugar level with energy bars or other stimulants. Many sugar-sensitive individuals will resort to caffeine, often drinking five or more cups of coffee per day to try to alleviate this feeling of chronic depression.

Researchers at the University of Sheffield in England found that diets low in fat increased an individual's sensitivity to pain. And when people were subjected to a higher fat diet, there was a significant decrease in their perception of pain.

The Serotonin Trap

Chocolate has been shown to be an effective, though short-term, mood elevator. Eating a chocolate bar can increase brain serotonin levels temporarily, while ridding you of depression and anxiety. However, the result does not last long. You may begin to crave chocolate on a more frequent basis because the result is so short-lived. Research published in the *British Journal of Clinical Psychology* studied women who reported an addiction to chocolate. The study concluded that in the long term, eating chocolate increased feelings of guilt, which lead to increased levels of depression and anxiety. They concluded that although chocolate is a food that provides immediate pleasure, the pleasure is short-lived and quickly followed by feelings of guilt and increased anxiety. The only solution is to eat a well-balanced diet and avoid processed, sugary foods.

Sugar Substitutes

The next time you crave a sugary food, try one or more of the following :60 second suggestions:

> **Protein:** Try eating some kind of protein instead. You will find that protein, combined with fresh fruits and vegetables, is the perfect antidote for sugar cravings.

> **Meditation:** Meditation is also an excellent antidote to anxiety and depression. Sit for a few minutes, quietly, using the *belly-chest-exhale technique*. If you focus on your breathing, you will find a tremendous sense of relaxation can block a craving for carbohydrates.

> **Exercise:** Exercise is an antidote for depression—taking a long

walk, lifting weights or practicing yoga or tai chi are but a few suggestions. Try using exercise rather than carbohydrates to elevate your mood.

Prayer: Pray for strength. Many people find prayer to be an antidote for depression. In fact, people who pray recover from surgery faster and are less prone to suicidal thoughts. :60 seconds of quiet prayer can work wonders.

Safe Mood Enhancers: St. John's Wort is an effective mood elevator. With your doctor's permission, try taking this supplement for six weeks and see if it helps your mood. It is safe and has far less side effects than antidepressant medication. However, this should be combined with a healthy diet, emphasizing protein and fruits and vegetables.

Therapy: Talk to a psychiatrist or a psychologist. It is possible that your depression may be due to an organic cause requiring medical and/or psychological intervention. Ask your doctor or friends for a referral to a qualified therapist.

:60 SECOND FOOD AND MOOD SUMMARY

- Fruits and vegetables are loaded with vitamins, minerals, trace elements and phytochemicals.
- Make breakfast and lunch your largest meals; dinner should be a light meal.
- Eat plenty of primitive foods and less new, processed foods.
- Research results suggest that low-fat diets can create increased anger and hostility.
- Low cholesterol could result in impulsive or violent behavior.
- Sugar-craving individuals may often feel depressed, sad or anxious.
- Try these fixes: increasing protein intake, meditating, exercising, praying, mood elevating and therapy if necessary.

Chapter 9

KEEPING HYDRATED

:60 Second Affirmation:
"Drinking fluids protects my health."

Sylvia, a charming thirty-eight-year-old librarian, originally came to see me for neck pain. She related to me that five years earlier she had both of her breasts removed due to cancer. I asked Sylvia about her dietary habits as a child and adult, looking for any hints of a cause for her cancer. I quizzed her for any family risk factors. Her lifestyle seemed admirable. She exercised regularly, ate a healthy diet, never smoked cigarettes and only occasionally drank coffee or tea. Not wanting to get sidetracked, I proceeded to treat her neck pain. Six months later she returned for a follow-up visit telling me she had cancer once again.

The story she told me was disturbing. Sylvia spent her entire youth in a small suburb of Miami, Florida, adjacent to a golf course. Her home bordered on the sixteenth hole near a large water trap the size of a small lake. She and her sister both supplemented their incomes by jumping into what looked like a swimming hole to retrieve golf balls which they sold back to the frustrated golfers. Her research into possible causes for her illness had revealed that this golf course was regularly sprayed with chemicals designed to keep the course green and lush. These chemicals were highly carcinogenic. She and her sister both developed breast cancer, as had many of the children in that neighborhood who were exposed to the spray or the water. Tragically, Sylvia died about nine months later after her breast cancer spread to her lungs and liver.

IS YOUR WATER SAFE?

The National Cancer Institute in Rockville, Maryland reported that children and adults can be exposed to potentially carcinogenic pesticides at home, in school, from lawns and gardens, through food and in contaminated drinking water. Water sprayed on crops may also be a contributing factor. They theorized that many types of cancers are probably due to pesticide exposure and appear to affect children even more than adults. Luckily, most of the drinking water in the United States and other European countries is generally safe. However, there are ways that you can protect yourself from the risk of disease by drinking pure and safe water.

There are many types of affordable water filters available. There is sufficient research to conclude that filtering your drinking water through some type of carbon filter, using a reverse osmosis unit, or distillation can increase the likelihood that you are drinking pure and healthy water. Although the vast majority of people have access to pure and safe drinking water, lead, copper, chlorine, aluminum and chemicals seeping into the groundwater from factories may have harmful side effects. Filtering your water is simply good preventative medicine for you and your children.

THE ESSENTIAL FLUID

In 1999, the University of Washington Nutritional Science Program concluded that many people are chronically dehydrated without knowing it. These researchers conjectured that this could be due to high consumption of caffeinated drinks and alcohol and exercising without replenishing lost fluids. They associated a deficiency in water or fluid intake with cancer, heart disease and kidney problems. They stated that the minimum water intake for adults should be approximately four to six cups per day. If possible, it is recommended to drink up to eight to ten cups of water a day.

The University of Iowa College of Medicine studied almost 800 teachers and found that those who drank less water had more than twice the number of infections than those who drank more water while working.

There is no question that what we drink is of major importance. All of our cells are continuously bathed in fluid. With insufficient liquid, our cells dry out and toxins build up, increasing the likelihood of contracting many types of diseases.

COFFEE OR TEA

There have been many experiments trying to link birth defects, cancer and heart disease to the intake of coffee or caffeine, but most of these experiments have been inconclusive. Although coffee does increase the secretion of acid in the stomach, there is no clear evidence linking it to stomach ulcers. However, once ulcers develop, people should be extra careful since coffee can often aggravate the symptoms. According to Dr. James Mills of the National Institute of Child Health and Human Development, most of the serious hazards that were initially linked to coffee "haven't panned out." However, women who drink caffeinated products do lose more calcium and should supplement their coffee drinking with a glass of milk for every two or three cups of coffee.

Some people are quite sensitive to the caffeine which is in coffee and do not realize it. While three to four cups of coffee per day may be a reasonable limit based upon the amount of caffeine, acids and oils in a cup of coffee, it is still possible to have an energy boost, as long as you do not drink coffee to excess. As the renaissance physician, Paracelsus said, "Nothing in itself is poison or cure, everything depends on the dosage."

Recent research has documented that, although coffee in moderate quantities is not harmful, many people who drink a lot of coffee typically engage in dangerous behaviors such as smoking cigarettes, eating unhealthy foods and leading a highly-stressed lifestyle. A high consumption of coffee is often a symptom that you have allowed too much stress to creep into your life. Cut down on the stress and often you will find less of a need to jump-start your nervous system every few hours with caffeine.

The Department of Public Health at Oregon State University concluded that beverages containing caffeine could aggravate premenstrual syndrome. The negative effects were apparent among both coffee and tea drinkers and were proportional to the amount of caffeine consumed. However, you can drink your morning cup of coffee without worry. Just try to avoid other beverages containing caffeine in large quantities or late in the day, as it may increase nervousness or the likelihood of insomnia.

TEA: A REJUVENATION STRATEGY

A recent study presented at the Second International Scientific Symposium on Tea and Human Health in Washington concluded that tea may also have value in preventing cancer. When their fifty-nine patients with pre-cancerous lesions drank or applied tea to their mouth, these lesions stopped growing and began to heal. Although this was a small study, other research also adds weight to the possibility that tea, especially green tea and black tea, may slow down the growth of other cancers as well. This is exciting, but more studies will need to be conducted to prove the efficacy of tea in helping combat some diseases.

Tea's origins date back to around 3000 B.C., and it was originally taken as a detoxifying medicine. Dutch traders first brought tea to Europe, but the British soon developed it as a prized commodity and transplanted it to India in the early 1800's. Since then, tea has become an integral part of the diet of many cultures around the world.

Flavinoids, possibly the primary medicinal components of tea, are non-vitamin antioxidants that appear to hinder chemicals that damage the body's cells. These damaged cells can mutate into cancer-causing genes and cholesterol that clogs the arteries of the heart. According to research at the University of Pennsylvania, the flavinoids in tea contain twenty to thirty times the antioxidant potency of Vitamins C and E. In animal studies, rats that drank black or green tea which then were exposed to carcinogens in tobacco developed fewer lung and throat tumors than rats that drank plain water. Mice which consume green tea develop fewer skin cancers when exposed to many hours of bright sunlight. A twenty-five-year-long study in Europe found that men who drank approximately five cups of tea had almost a seventy percent lower risk of stroke than men who drank less.

Green tea in moderate amounts has no known toxic side effects. It is a mild stimulant and contains only half the caffeine in your typical cup of coffee. Two cups of green tea have the Vitamin C equal to one cup of orange juice and enough fluoride to prevent cavities. In our modern world, where we are bombarded by pesticides, tobacco smoke, air pollutants and stress, green tea may be an important antidote. One reason why people living in Japan may have lower blood fat and a lower incidence of heart disease may be because they favor green tea over coffee.

Green tea is one of the world's oldest beverages. Thus, it fits well into the *:60 Second Rejuvenation Strategy* because it is like the primitive, unprocessed food used by our ancient ancestors. But there are a number of different types of tea and the choices can be confusing. Tea comes from an evergreen shrub that thrives in tropical and semi-tropical climates. Green tea is the least processed, youngest and freshest of all of the types of tea. The green tea leaves are steamed, rolled and dried, while other teas are fermented.

SO, WHAT SHOULD I DO?

Drinking plenty of water is one of the most effective ways of flushing harmful toxins from the body. Pure, fresh water is a very important part of a healthy lifestyle. Try drinking a cup of water right after, or even with, your next cup of coffee. You will still be able to drink your favorite beverage, but at the same time you will keep your body properly hydrated. Or drink a glass of water twice a day, as if you were taking a medication. Remember, pure water can prevent many diseases and should not be overlooked.

However, because coffee apparently does not possess the same healthy characteristics as green or black tea, try to avoid drinking coffee all day long. Instead, have a cup of green tea in the afternoon when you desire a quick pick-me-up. Black tea possesses many of the same benefits as green tea. It may be taken with some milk and will provide a delicious alternative to coffee.

:60 SECOND FLUID SUGGESTIONS SUMMARY

- Adults should drink a minimum of four to six cups of water per day.
- Filtering your drinking water is good preventative medicine.
- Women who drink caffeinated products lose more calcium and should supplement their coffee drinking with a glass of milk for every two or three cups of coffee.
- Try to avoid any beverage containing caffeine in large quantities or late in the day, as it may increase nervousness or the likelihood of insomnia.
- Medical research is concluding that drinking green tea may actually lower the risk of cancers and some other diseases.

Chapter 10

HERBS—DESIGNER VEGETABLES

:60 Second Affirmation:
"In sickness and in health, nature protects me."

Tony's parents were delighted when he graduated from Stanford University with a Ph.D. in computer science and business. They assumed he would soon be making his fortune working for one of Silicon Valley's top companies.

Since an early age, Tony had suffered from a minor heart disorder called atrial fibrillation. At irregular intervals, his heart would skip a beat and then race out of control for a few seconds. As a child he feared that his heart would stop beating and he would die. Tony also had asthma which, without warning, would flare-up badly, necessitating a trip with his worried parents to the emergency room. One of his doctors suggested that young Tony study a musical instrument, like the clarinet or saxophone, to strengthen his lungs. Tony liked the suggestion.

He enjoyed playing the saxophone and continued to play with local clubs in his well-rehearsed jazz quartet throughout college and graduate school. Although he was still a straight "A" student in computer science, his only real passion in life was playing jazz saxophone. After graduation, just as his parents hoped, the job offers poured in. Tony shocked his parents by rejecting all of them. He told them that he decided to become a full time jazz musician.

One day, while bicycling to his rehearsal studio, a drunk driver swerved into him, throwing him off his bike. Fortunately, he was not seriously hurt, but he had sustained whiplash with serious cuts and bruises over his arms and legs.

He came to me a few weeks later complaining of a stiff, aching neck. After six sessions of massage, mobilization and a home stretching routine, Tony recovered completely. However, he also complained that his heart and lung problems had worsened—probably due to the emotional stress following the accident. I prescribed three herbs for him, Hawthorn, Thyme and Elecampane. Hawthorn is an excellent heart remedy because it is able to either speed up or slow down the heart rate and Elecampane and Thyme both improve lung function.

After taking Hawthorn for six months, Tony no longer suffered any palpitations. His lungs had improved significantly, and he rarely needed to use medication. Even after he stopped taking his heart and lung herbs, he has not had a relapse for over a year. Although it is possible that he will need to take Hawthorn again in the future, Tony considers himself cured.

Now he is taking herbs on a regular basis. Colds are treated with echinacea and garlic, he takes kava kava to relax and is avidly studying herbal medicine. Tony plans to enter medical school in the fall to become a naturopathic physician. He has cut his second jazz album and plans to use the profits to help support his naturopathic studies. Tony now wants to serenade his audience with jazz music and herbal medicine.

USING HERBS WISELY

Herbal therapies are growing in popularity due to their gentle, but effective action. Medical doctors throughout the world rely upon herbal medicine for many conditions. When taking herbal supplements, follow a few simple guidelines:

1. Always take one dose (one herb at a time) and then wait three to four hours prior to taking more. During this waiting period, you can assess if you suffer any type of allergic reaction to the herb's active ingredients. Never continue to take an herb if you have any type of negative reaction. Rashes, stomach upset and headache are a few of the symptoms you may experience if you are allergic to an herbal preparation.

2. Teas are the safest form of herbal therapy but are often less effective than stronger capsules, tablets or liquid tinctures. The average amount of herb in a capsule is usually between 300 and 500 milligrams of powdered root or leaf. However, capsules are available in a variety of sizes, so dosage may vary. When in doubt, always follow the directions on the label. If a range of dosages is given, always start with the lowest dose. If symptoms persist, worsen or become serious, consult your physician.

3. Women usually require lower doses than men and smaller, lighter individuals should take less than a heavier person. Children require lower doses than adults.

HERBS FOR COMMON CONDITIONS

1. *Allergies:* Nettle and goldenseal.
2. *Colds and Flu:* Echinacea, goldenseal and garlic.
3. *Exhaustion or General Imbalance:* Ginseng and siberian ginseng.
4. *Female/Menstrual and Hormonal Irregularities:* Chaste berry (or vitex) and black cohosh.
5. *Male/Prostate Problems:* Saw palmetto.
6. *Psychological Problems and Anxiety:* St. John's wort, kava kava and valerian.

If you would like to use herbal therapy in your *:60 Second Rejuvenation Strategy,* the following list is a good place to start. They are all extremely effective and safe when used properly. *Note: Always consult your physician before using herbal remedies to ascertain whether you may have some counterindication or whether mixing these substances with each other or other medications could be harmful to your health. Dosages listed below are general guidelines; carefully read the labels on every product you buy and follow those dosage instructions.*

THE TOP TEN HERBS

1. **Chaste berry (or vitex):** Chaste berry or vitex has its greatest use in normalizing the activity of female sex hormones. Thus, it is quite effective for pre-menstrual syndrome, as an aid to menopausal changes or to relieve other problems associated with menstruation. Results may be obtained after one to two months, but it is not unusual to require six to twelve months for a complete cure. It may be combined with black cohosh for menstrual problems. Available in liquid or capsule form, take between 200 and 250 milligrams two times a day or as directed on the package.

2. **Echinacea:** This is a common garden plant that enhances the immune system and improves the body's resistance to infection of all kinds, particularly colds and flu. Echinacea is taken as soon as cold or flu symptoms appear; a small dose combined

with goldenseal every two to three hours at the first sign of an infection is adequate. For more severe cold and flu symptoms, take up to 1,000 milligrams a day of this combination (echinacea plus goldenseal) until relief is achieved. You may take between 200 and 300 milligrams per day a few weeks on and a few weeks off throughout the year to help strengthen your immune system. Cycling on and off herbs can prevent your body from becoming accustomed to them, which would eventually limit their effectiveness.

3. **Garlic:** Garlic is a member of the onion family and is a well-established remedy for hardening of the arteries, upper respiratory infections, high cholesterol and infections almost anywhere in the body, especially the lungs and intestines. Deodorized garlic capsules are available in most health food stores, pharmacies and even supermarkets. Take 200 to 300 milligrams each day to prevent colds, flu and infections or combine with echinacea and goldenseal as an effective therapy for almost all types of colds, flu and infections. If you are more daring, try taking approximately one-half clove of raw garlic three times per day in place of the capsules (or as directed on the package). It may be cut up into small pieces and placed in a salad, on a sandwich or swallowed with a small amount of water. When taking raw garlic, eating parsley will disguise most of the odor.

4. **Ginseng and Siberian Ginseng:** Ginseng is one of the oldest medicinal herbs in Asia and has been touted for its ability to create miraculous cures. It is primarily used as a general tonic and mild stimulant which can treat fatigue, over exertion and general weakness. It is quite effective at improving physical and mental capacity in the elderly and can even relieve mild depression. A less expensive and more easily available substitute for ginseng is a plant called siberian ginseng or eleutherococcus. If you're feeling rundown, try taking 200 milligrams of either herb twice per day for one month or as directed on the package. If you suffer from any serious emotional complaints, take these herbs only under the supervision of a qualified doctor or herbalist.

5. **Goldenseal:** Goldenseal is one of our most useful remedies and has a function similar to many antibiotics. It has demonstrated effectiveness against many types of bacteria, viruses and

fungi. It is especially helpful for upper respiratory infections, such as most colds and flu, as well as allergies. Take 200 to 300 milligrams two to three times a day for a maximum of two weeks or as directed on the package. Goldenseal is especially effective as a supplement when combined with echinacea and garlic to treat almost all types of colds, flu and systemic infections.

6. ***Kava Kava:*** Kava kava was originally called *intoxicating pepper* and was a popular drink among South Pacific Islanders for special guests and royalty. Detailed investigations of this herb have noted that most people feel calm and relaxed with enhanced mental activity. It has become a very popular antidote for nervous depression and anxiety. Although valerian may provide a stronger sedating effect, kava kava also has mild antidepressant properties, making it a great all-around antidote for many kinds of psychological difficulties. If you are feeling stressed, take a 200 to 300 milligram capsule each hour until you feel more relaxed. If the stressful situation lasts for more than a day, take a capsule twice a day for up to one week or as directed on the package.

7. ***Nettle:*** Nettle or stinging nettle strengthens and supports the whole body. Throughout Europe, nettle is often used as a spring tonic. It is extremely beneficial for allergies and helps to relieve watery eyes, itching and other symptoms caused by pollen allergies. It is quite effective in this regard when combined with goldenseal. To relieve hayfever symptoms, take a 200 to 300 milligram capsule twice a day just before pollen season arrives. For acute symptoms, take two to three capsules twice daily or as directed on the package.

8. ***St. John's Wort:*** St. John's wort derives its name from the fact that it begins to flower around St. John's tide, the summer solstice at the end of June. It has become quite popular because it is very effective at treating mild to moderate depression. Although some improvement in mood may be achieved after two to three weeks, it is necessary to take St. John's wort for two to three months prior to evaluating its total effect. Take St. John's wort with kava kava when the depression is also associated with anxiety. Take 200 to 300 milligrams two to three times per day or as directed on the package.

9. *Saw Palmetto:* Saw palmetto grows wild in Mediterranean countries and Eastern North America. Recent investigations by physicians and researchers document its effectiveness at relieving the symptoms associated with a swollen or inflamed prostate. In fact, many medical doctors are now prescribing saw palmetto rather than medication. Take 200 milligrams two to three times each day or as directed on the package.

10. *Valerian:* Valerian is a powerful sedative, mainly used to treat anxiety and sleeplessness. However, it should not be used when there is depression because it can aggravate the problem. Combining valerian with passionflower and/or hops may improve its effectiveness. Take up to 500 milligrams one half hour before bedtime or as directed on the package.

:60 SECOND HERBAL REMEDIES SUMMARY

- Always consult your physician and pharmacist before taking any herbal remedy. This is especially important for those taking prescription medication.
- Take one dose of only one herb and wait for three to four hours in order to assess your reaction to the herb. Then, if you experience no negative reactions, take the herb for one week before introducing another.
- Consult an herbalist if possible for advice on which herbal remedies are best for you.

Chapter 11

TIME—THE TEMPTING TRAP

:60 Second Affirmation:
"My inner clock knows the time."

Samantha rose to prominence in the literary world by publishing a popular series of natural health cookbooks. She had a wonderful marriage, three lovely teenage girls and a stunning home overlooking San Francisco Bay. She had no financial problems. In fact, in addition to her house, she had investments in stocks and bonds which totaled more than a million dollars. In spite of a happy family, an overflowing bank account and a supportive husband, she was unable to sleep.

Her room had thick curtains over the windows to prevent the tiniest sliver of light from announcing that dawn had arrived. Her husband's tossing and turning became an irritant, so she asked him to sleep in the guest room down the hall. Samantha's physician had prescribed numerous medications which were somewhat helpful. However, she became fearful of their long-term addictive side effects. Before too long, taking pills had become a regular habit. She finally threw the pills away when she found herself steadily, over time, increasing the dosage.

Before Thomas Edison developed the light bulb, we were forced to follow the rhythms of nature. When it was dark, we were forced to slow down. Even with candles, a dimly lit house encouraged a slower, less active lifestyle. By adding light bulbs to our lives, we transformed the tranquillity of evening into a stimulating event. Now a typical evening may be punctuated with bright lights, television sets, the glare of a computer screens and responding to pagers, e-mail messages or cell phones. Evening no longer allows us respite from all the stimulation of a busy day.

Primitive man was very busy during the day. After all, with nightfall he was forced to deal with his inability to move around safely because he was surrounded by darkness and unseen dangers. He would use every bit of sunlight possible, knowing that evening was a time for rest, not productivity. By placing a stick in the ground, he could manufacture a simple sundial and then plan his day accordingly. There was no need to be precise—being a few minutes off here or there was not a serious problem. Man eventually used the bells in the church tower or the blowing of a steam whistle of a factory to mark important times of the day.

However, the advent of the railroad made these bells and whistles an inexact source of timekeeping. As the railroad spanned continents, it became important to meet the train at a precise location at the appropriate time. Prior to the invention of the train, a slight delay in most things was not a serious dilemma. However, anxious passengers on a full train did not want to wait fifteen to twenty minutes for someone to saunter up to the train station loaded with baggage. The advent of the train created a universal need for people coast to coast to synchronize their watches. Light bulbs and trains converted man from being sensitive to the light and dark cycle, to a race driven by the unstoppable pace of civilization.

In 1989, researcher Stefania Folline spent almost four months alone in a cave, thirty feet below the New Mexico desert. She was isolated from civilization, without sunlight or a clock to demarcate day and night. Stefania experienced the same type of rhythm common to all volunteers who placed themselves in isolation, free from the constraints of timekeeping. Stefania lost track of time and began sleeping about once every twenty-eight hours. Numerous other experiments like this have produced slightly different time cycles, but there is one thing the participants all shared in common. They all produced a natural *biological rhythm* of their own, even without the influence of clocks, lightbulbs or the natural light/dark cycle. These types of experiments are proof that human beings possess their own internal clock.

THE RHYTHMS OF NATURE

Our hearts beat approximately once every second. Meanwhile, the cerebral spinal fluid which flows through our brain and spinal cord ebbs and flows approximately eight to twelve times per minute. Every minute, our stomach creates ripples of peristalsis, moving food through our digestive tract. Ten to fifteen times every minute we unconsciously inhale and then exhale. Our body is composed of a marvelous symphony of rhythms inextricably tied to our cells, hormones and nervous system.

Women will testify that their monthly menstrual cycle has a strong influence upon their awareness of the passage of time. Every month pre-menopausal women notice real psychological and physiological changes and then menstruate like clockwork. At regular intervals, both men and women are being driven by hormonal fluctuations, like great high and low tides. Almost everyone has experienced those late afternoon yawns that occur almost every day an hour or two after lunch. This waxing and waning of our energy cycle is a direct result of our complex biological rhythm.

MORNING RUSH, AFTERNOON SLUMP

Medical researchers have discovered that most heart attacks occur on Monday mornings. That is the time most individuals, still slightly groggy from a deep night's sleep, too hurriedly try to jump-start their metabolism to begin their work day. This could be one reason why most schools of meditation encourage their students to meditate in the morning. It is an important time to become more physiologically attuned to our natural rhythm, rather than the more socially encouraged cup of coffee in morning rush hour traffic.

Many of us eat a very skimpy breakfast. We grab a few vitamins with whatever food is quickly consumed, wash breakfast down with a few gulps of coffee, grab our papers or briefcase and run for the car. Yet, research has shown this is both illogical and unhealthy behavior. Children who eat a full breakfast have been shown to be more attentive than those who grab a quick candy bar or doughnut and run for the school bus. In experiments that allowed people to only eat one meal per day, those who only ate breakfast lost weight; while many who ate only dinner gained weight.

Regardless of our bad habits, as the morning wears on, we still may feel energetic, powered by our body's natural early morning productive rhythm. When lunchtime arrives, we grab a quick hamburger, french fries and a chocolate milkshake. Still feeling energized, we return to work ready to attack the stack of papers on our desk begging for attention. But then, about one to two hours later, we are hit by the afternoon slump. Afraid of falling asleep, we hurriedly grab a cup or two of coffee to avoid this late afternoon letdown. Enlivened by our caf-feine jolt, we finish our work and head for home.

After dinner, our bodies begin to slow down and our body tem-perature (which has been rising throughout the day) begins to cool. Our bodies are preparing to go to sleep. As melatonin begins to filter through our bloodstream, our heart rate and blood pressure slow, and we begin to prepare for bed.

UPSETTING THE CYCLE

As the evening approaches, many of us respond to our slowing rhythm and try to unwind. However, with our ever-increasing work pressure or with a late night phone call or check of our e-mail, we can actually dis-tort our own natural rhythm. Watching an exciting movie or the news until 11:00 or 12:00 at night, we stimulate our bodies into thinking it is actually morning. Then, after plopping into bed around midnight, we are rudely awakened by our 6:00 A.M. alarm clock, again throwing us outside our natural rhythm.

Our ancestors were required to slow down in the winter. After all, a three-foot snowfall would prevent primitive man from even dashing a few yards in any direction. Without the long summer days to allow fren-zied hunting and gathering activity, winter was a time of rest. Similarly, animals display a hibernation strategy and slow down during the winter to conserve energy during this quiet period. Yet three feet of snow does not stop the daring New Yorker from charging off at 7:00 A.M. to get the subway or race down the local expressway—his car well outfitted with a powerful heater and snow tires. Although this New Yorker may be on time for his morning business meeting, often he may feel anxious or angry, subconsciously feeling out of sync with the short days and long nights. This lack of sunlight can also create serious depression in some individuals. An estimated ten million Americans suffer from Seasonal Affective Disorder (SAD) and researchers suspect that another twenty-five million may experience some SAD symptoms, including weight gain, mild depression, lethargy and carbohydrate or sugar cravings.

In the autumn or early winter, many people with SAD begin to feel listless and rundown. But unfortunately, many of them do not asso-ciate their depression with a lack of sunlight. Instead, many individuals seek out antidepressants during the winter. They are quite pleased to notice their improved mood in the spring and summer. Little do they know that the reason for their improved mood is the longer days and shorter nights.

Many parents, myself included, watch their teenagers stay up late, talking on the telephone or playing stimulating computer games. A syndrome called Delayed Sleep Phase Syndrome (DSPS) causes a delay in the normal sleep cycle of teenagers. Teens suffering from DSPS note that sleep comes on later and later, eventually creating an inability to get to bed at a reasonable hour. Yet bright and early each morning they are awakened by their alarm clock telling them it is time to go to school. This can cause increasing *sleep debt* with concomitant lower achievement in school and problems concentrating.

Few things are more disturbing to our inner sense of time than the jarring effects of jet lag. Flying into another time zone causes our bodies to be out of sync with our natural biological rhythm and our own light/dark cycle. There are very few proven remedies for jet lag. One of the more effective natural cures is the dietary supplement melatonin. It has been shown that taking melatonin before bedtime helps induce sleep and restores our natural biological rhythm. Another suggestion is to get outside as much as possible during the day and exposing yourself to daylight. We set our internal clocks by the light/dark cycle of our hemisphere. Thus, when you travel to a foreign country, try spending as many hours as possible outside, allowing your body to adapt to this new light/dark schedule.

TIME AND THE REJUVENATION STRATEGY

There are many things you can do to reacquaint yourself with your natural biological rhythm. Try the following :60 second strategies:

1. *Decide if you are a morning or evening person.* Being in touch with your natural rhythm is the first step. Observe your natural rhythm during holidays, on weekends and during long vacations. Try to plan your work life, if possible, around your natural energy schedule. If you are a morning person, try to plan most of your intensive work for the early morning hours. If you are an afternoon or evening person, that is the time for important business meetings.

2. *Try to eat a large breakfast and lunch and a light dinner.* Research indicates that breakfast and lunch are your most important meals. These meals give your body the energy it needs to complete a full day's work and elevate body temperature and increase one's ability to perform physical activities which burns

up calories. Eating late at night will only disrupt your sleep cycle and encourage weight gain.

3. *Get plenty of sunlight.* Even if you work inside of a building all day, try to get outside during the afternoon. This exposure to sunlight can improve your mood, reduce jet lag when you are traveling, harmonize your inner biological clock to the light/dark cycle and help reduce stress.

4. *Follow seasonal cycles.* Just as you should be busier during the day and slower at night, try to plan to be busier during the late spring, summer and early fall—lightening your schedule during the winter. This will harmonize your biological rhythm with the rhythms of nature.

5. *Slow down in the evening.* After dinner, try to unwind and avoid highly stimulating activities. This does not mean you cannot go out and party on Saturday night, but most of your evenings should be quiet, allowing your body to be in harmony with nature.

:60 SECOND NATURAL RHYTHM SUMMARY

• Try to plan your work life around your natural energy cycle.
• Breakfast and lunch are the most important meals; late night meals encourage weight gain and contribute to insomnia.
• Exposure to sunlight can harmonize your inner biological clock to the light/dark cycle, help reduce stress and depression and reduce jet lag.
• Follow seasonal cycles—plan to be busier in the late spring, summer and early fall and lighten your schedule during the winter.

Chapter 12

SLEEP—UNCONSCIOUS MEDITATION

:60 Second Affirmation:
"With each breath, my rest becomes deeper."

Corinne was plagued by chronic headaches. Tired of gulping down fistfuls of ibuprofen, she consulted her family doctor, asking for advice. Her doctor sent her to a neurologist. Following x-rays, an MRI and an intense neurological work-up, she was pronounced healthy with no abnormal signs or symptoms. Her anxiety about her headaches was heightened because of her history of breast cancer. Three years earlier she had a partial mastectomy. She worried that her headaches could be a symptom of metastatic cancer.

I examined her and found tremendous tightness in her upper back and neck. After giving her some basic advice regarding posture and exercise, I proceeded to loosen up her tight muscles and bones. However, following five treatments, there was no improvement. She still complained of chronic neck pain and headaches. We spent some time discussing her problem and she revealed a new fact: her headaches and neck pain were worse in the morning.

Corinne originally thought her headaches and neck pain occurred all the time, but as her neck muscles loosened, she realized that the pain was significantly more intense upon awakening. I concluded that there was a problem with how she was sleeping. She told me that she had difficulty relaxing and falling asleep and that she always slept on her side using a feather pillow to support her *head. I first suggested some minor lifestyle changes that would help prepare her body for sleep. I also explained to her that it is virtually impossible to maintain proper neck posture while sleeping on your side with a feather pillow. I taught her what type of pillow was most beneficial when sleeping on one's side. Once she implemented the minor lifestyle changes and began using a more supportive pillow, she began sleeping better and her headaches and neck pain dissipated.*

THE SLEEPY SOCIETY

Modern life bombards us with stimulation. Television sets, cell phones, radios and pagers are constantly reminding us to stay alert. Even the electric light bulb, a relatively recent invention, can be an obstacle to good sleep.

Researchers at both Stanford Medical Center and the University of Oregon have concluded that bright light can trick our brains into thinking that we should be awake and alert. The importance of this fact cannot be underestimated. The simple acts of watching television late at night, keeping your house well lit prior to going to bed and checking your e-mail in the evening can all have the effect of jump-starting your metabolism. Our early ancestors did not have these impediments to sleep. *Homo sapiens* living 50,000 to 100,000 years ago did not have houses with dark shades to avert morning sunlight, nor did they have light bulbs and e-mail to stimulate them in the evening. Consequently, their biological clocks were constantly being tuned to the systematic dark and light cycle of the earth's changing seasons, which was beyond their control. Although it is impossible to gauge the sleeplessness of our ancestors, we do know that sleep problems are becoming much more frequent as we approach the 21st century. Even as recently as the 1800s, people had markedly fewer sleep disorders.

Researchers at Laval University in Quebec looked at the data from more than a dozen treatment studies of patients with difficulty sleeping. They concluded that sleep habits could be easily improved, reducing the need for medication.

WHY SLEEP?

Researchers at Carnegie Mellon University and the University of Pennsylvania found that the amount and quality of sleep actually effects how sick people get. The immune system is the body's primary defense against viruses and bacteria that invade the body, causing disease. This mounting evidence that sleep may help strengthen the immune system is quite important. A good night's sleep must be considered an integral part of any rejuvenation strategy. But how do you know if you are getting enough sleep?

William Dement, M.D., one of the world's foremost authorities on sleep, terms the physical condition of lacking enough sleep, *sleep debt*. Dement feels that the simplest way to measure sleep debt is to assess your daytime sleepiness. If you feel sleepy more than a couple of times during the day, you may be suffering some type of sleep debt.

:60 SECOND SLEEP IMPROVING TIPS

There are a number of things you can do to sleep better. Most of them involve simple changes to your lifestyle, rather than the need for herbs or medication. First, try the following :60 second suggestions:

1. *Sleeping Tools:* Choose the right bed and pillows. If you awaken in the morning with back pain, you are probably sleeping in the wrong bed. If you awaken with neck pain, you probably need to change your pillow. I will discuss in detail later in this chapter the best pillow and mattress options. Being too warm, too cold or hindered by the wrong type of quilt or comforter can also disturb your sleep. It is very important that you pay attention to all of these details. Your bed needs to be your most comfortable place on earth. After all, you will spend approximately one-third of your life there.

2. *Sleeping Environment:* Be certain that your room is an ideal environment for sleep. Notice how you feel with the windows open or closed. Some people prefer a cooler or a warmer environment. It is very important that your room block noise and light from disturbing your sleep. Primitive man never had to worry about the honking horns from taxi cabs or the roar of an overhead jet plane, but you may need to close your window, turn on a fan or buy a white noise maker to quiet your environment.

3. *Bedtime Ritual:* Establish a bedtime ritual. Some people find gentle yoga stretching to be calming and helpful to induce sleep. Other people find that reading a book (as long as it is not a chilling murder mystery) is also an effective sleep-inducer. Taking a warm bath, dimming the lights an hour

before bedtime and avoiding stimulation will all help induce a good night's sleep.

4. **Regular Bedtime:** Establish a regular bedtime. Research indicates that going to sleep at the same time every night is a tremendous aid to a good night's sleep. All of your body's chemicals and hormones gradually learn an established pattern and will trigger to prepare you for sleep if you follow a daily ritual.

5. **Food and Drink:** Be certain to avoid coffee, tea, soda, chocolate or medications that include caffeine in the evening. Many people report that drinking alcohol also disturbs their sleep. Although having one or two drinks with dinner may be very relaxing, it can also make it more difficult to sleep. Be sure that you finish your evening meal a few hours before retiring and try to eat a light dinner. Overeating late in the day can make you feel uncomfortable and deprive you of a good night's sleep since your body will go into overdrive to digest all that food.

6. **Stimulation:** Avoid stimulation at least one hour before bedtime. Watching television, checking your e-mail, having a fight with your spouse or anything that does not involve some type of unwinding can be a hindrance to a good night's sleep. Remember that *Homo sapiens* evolved with the ability to adapt to a night and day or light/dark cycle. Be certain that you avoid any heavy stimulation, especially bright lights, in the evening.

7. **Exercise:** It is best to exercise vigorously during the day. A brisk walk that only requires a few minutes can actually prove to be an antidote to sleeplessness. Exercising during the day while exposing yourself to sunlight and then slowing down in the evening while dimming the lights in your home will help reset your internal clock and put you more in tune with natural rhythms.

Melatonin

Melatonin is a hormone secreted by the pineal gland that tells the brain that it is dark outside. Long, cold winter nights tell the body to secrete more melatonin, and short summer nights lead to lower levels. Even very low doses—up to 0.5 milligrams—can modify your biological clock, telling your brain that it is time to go to sleep. Melatonin can be purchased in pill form as a sleep aid. However, because it is a new supplement, check with your doctor before taking melatonin. There is some concern that it could be harmful for people with heart problems.

Herbs

There are many herbs that help induce sleep: valerian, chamomile, passionflower and oats are very common herbal remedies to improve sleep. Generally, a few capsules or droppers full, thirty to sixty minutes before bedtime, will make it easier to fall asleep and help you sleep a bit longer. However, always check the dosage recommended by the manufacturer.

Medication

If you are still having trouble sleeping after having tried these behavioral suggestions and herbs, check with your doctor to see if medication is appropriate for you.

Studies have shown that heightened states of anxiety during the day can produce an increase in insomnia. Researchers at San Jose State University studied college students and concluded that concern about time was highly correlated with sleep problems.

THE TWILIGHT ZONE

We have all experienced the state of *twilight sleep*, being half-asleep and half-awake. It is quite similar to the psychological state obtained during deep meditation. You will find that meditating in bed, just after waking up, is very easy, even if you have failed trying to meditate many times.

Morning Meditation

Even if you have never meditated, try meditating for :60 seconds upon awakening. It is quite simple if you follow these easy steps:

1. Don't start thinking. Try lying on your back, with your knees bent and your feet flat on the bed. Stay under the covers where you are warm and comfortable. Place your arms at your sides

or interlock your hands on your belly. If you desire to change positions, do so very slowly and gently. You can meditate in whatever position feels most comfortable for you. If you feel more comfortable lying on your side, spend a short time on one side and then roll onto the other side.

2. Always breathe into the belly first. Use the belly-chest-exhale breathing technique.

3. When thoughts arise, don't pay attention to them. It is okay to look at them, but don't focus on them. Whenever you observe thoughts, turn your attention back to your belly-chest-exhale breathing pattern.

4. After you have spent :60 seconds meditating, get up and start your day.

5. Try to bring the calm from your meditation into your morning routine. Try to avoid stress or excessive stimulation until you have had at least five to fifteen minutes of time to transition from your twilight sleep meditation back to the real world.

SLEEPING, PILLOWS AND BEDS

If you have headaches and/or neck pain in the morning, it is probably caused by a problem with your pillow or bed. If you get pain later in the day, it is probably due to daily life activity.

The world is divided into four kinds of sleepers: side sleepers, back sleepers, stomach sleepers and rock-and-rollers. If you almost always sleep on either your side, back or stomach, it is very easy to design a bed and pillow combination which will work well for you. If you are a rock-and-roller and you toss and turn all through the night, you will require a more complex arrangement.

:60 Second Side Sleeper Strategy

The vast majority of people find sleeping on their side the most comfortable position. Yet most people use a pillow that is far too low. When the pillow does not support the head sufficiently to maintain a straight spine, the head will sink toward the bed, scrunching up the head, neck and shoulders which can create pinched nerves and compressed neck disks. The most important solution is to raise the pillow you sleep on.

Try lying on your side with your head on the pillow. Does your head sink down or is it in alignment with the rest of your spine? If you are uncertain, stand up and note the relationship of your head to your neck and shoulders. Then lie down on your side again, maintaining this posture. If your head tilts toward the bed, your pillow is too low. Try adding another pillow or raising your pillow by placing folded towels or blankets underneath it until you feel comfortable. By raising and lowering your pillow you will be able to experience the most comfortable angle for your head and neck.

If you enjoy the feeling of a feather pillow, but prefer sleeping on your side, you may need to place a piece of foam underneath your feather pillow in order to elevate it to the proper height. Or you can purchase a more supportive pillow from your local department store, a back shop or other store that specializes in orthopedic products.

:60 Second Back Sleeper Strategy

People who sleep on their backs usually require a lower pillow than those who sleep on their sides. The space between the head and bed is quite a bit larger when you are on your side than on your back. If you prefer to sleep on your back, you may be content with a feather pillow but may need a more supportive or higher pillow, especially if your head juts forward. Lie on your back and try the same exercise which we did in the side sleeping position. Raise and lower your pillow, using foam, towels or blankets, until you find the most comfortable position for your head. This is your ideal back sleeping posture.

:60 Second Stomach Sleeper Strategy

Ideally, you should not sleep on your stomach. Sleeping on your stomach forces you to twist your neck into a very contorted position. However, some people cannot sleep any other way. Some people feel very emotionally vulnerable with their stomach and chest exposed to the world. If you must sleep on your stomach, you should not use any pillow. If possible, try using a position halfway between side sleeping and stomach sleeping. You can achieve this position by lying on your side and then half rolling onto your stomach with your top leg bent towards your chest. If you like the half-lying position, it is an ideal substitute for the stomach position because it provides less stress on your head and neck.

Stomach sleepers often prefer a pillow that is lower than a side sleeper. If you find the half-lying position to be uncomfortable, try raising and lowering your pillow, using foam, towels or a blanket until you find your ideal head position.

:60 Second Rock and Roller Strategy

If you move from side to back to stomach throughout the night, you will require a more complex sleeping arrangement. Ideally, you need an orthopedic pillow. These pillows often are higher around the edges and lower in the center. This allows you to roll onto your side to lie on the higher portion of the pillow and then roll onto your back to lower your head into the depression of the pillow.

Finding a Comfortable Bed

Many of my patients are surprised or sometimes depressed when I tell them that they spend one-third of their lives in bed. However, that is the truth. Therefore, your bed is a very important part of your life and a key component in creating a happy and healthy life.

The bed which you find most comfortable will be dependent upon your shape. If you are pear shaped or shaped like a triangle, you will find a very firm bed with a soft top will be most effective. The soft top will allow your shoulders or hips to sink slightly into the bed, allowing your spine to maintain its neutral posture. If your bed is too hard, put one or two inches of soft foam on top of your mattress and see if that improves your sleeping position. If your body is straight and lacks curves, you will probably feel most comfortable on a firm, supportive mattress.

Buying a new bed is a complicated process because there are so many choices available. No matter what type of bed you decide to purchase, always buy one that seems too hard for you. If you buy a bed that is too soft, it is impossible to make it more supportive. However, if the bed is too hard, you only need to add one to two inches of soft foam to the top.

Most people find that a standard box spring and mattress is ideal. When you are shopping for a mattress, you should spend at least five minutes lying on the bed. This can feel like an eternity. Most people who choose the wrong mattress lie on it for five or ten seconds, never truly assessing whether or not it fits their needs. If you feel embarrassed spending this much time on the mattress in a store, make sure your bed has a guarantee allowing you to return it after a minimum of one week. It is often impossible to know the appropriateness of a mattress without spending at least a few days testing it.

An alternative suggestion to buying a mattress and box spring is to purchase only the mattress and place it on top of a platform. Because a platform is firmer than a box spring it will provide more support and reduce the money you spend on your bed—you will never need to buy a box spring again.

Another option is a water bed. Water beds come in many styles and sizes. While some individuals swear by their warmth and comfort, others dislike them because they find them too soft and difficult to get in and out of. If you are thinking about buying a water bed, be sure to test them out to see if you feel comfortable laying down on one and getting up from one. If you decide to buy a water bed, be certain to choose the waveless variety. Waveless water beds are composed of baffles that make the bed much firmer and more comfortable.

If you like a firm bed, you might try a Japanese futon. This is often sold as a folding bed made of cotton or foam and is usually placed on a platform rather than a bed frame. Usually, these can be conveniently folded up during the day and used as a chair or sofa, then pulled out in the evening to be used as a bed. The ideal futon is a four or five inch foam mattress called a "shikibuton" with a separate, one inch cotton pad on top called the "futon."

Once you have mastered the proper pillow and head position and purchased the appropriate mattress, you are ready for a good night's sleep. Remember to keep the room at a comfortable temperature and do not spend long hours in bed if you are having trouble sleeping. Try to avoid heavy eating before bed, do not drink caffeinated beverages and shun rigorous exercise. Some gentle stretching, a warm bath or some herbal tea will prepare you for a good night's sleep. Your bed needs to be your quiet refuge from the storms of daily life. If you are having trouble sleeping, get up and read a boring book—the dictionary, or a technical manual. Surely this will drive you promptly back to bed and to a good night's sleep!

:60 SECOND SLEEP STRATEGY SUMMARY

- Research has shown that bright light can trick our brains into thinking we should be awake and alert, and heightened states of anxiety during the day can produce an increase in insomnia.

- Other research indicates that sleep actually affects how sick people get.
- There are a number of things you can do to sleep better; most involve simple changes to your lifestyle rather than the need for herbs or medication.
- Try meditation upon awakening in the morning, while you are still in your twilight sleep.
- If you have headaches, back pain or neck pain in the morning, it is probably caused by a problem with your pillow and/or bed.
- If you get pain later in the day, it is probably due to daily life activity.
- Determine whether you are a side, back or stomach sleeper—or a rock-and-roller.
- Always buy a bed that seems too hard for you, as you can always add a soft top or piece of foam.
- Avoid stimulation before bedtime.
- To induce sleep, try activities that promote relaxation or boredom.

PART 3

APPLYING
:60 SECOND STRATEGIES
TO EVERYDAY LIFE

Chapter 13

BUSINESS BODY LANGUAGE—
HEALTHY BUSINESS BEHAVIOR

:60 Second Affirmation:
"I develop my strength, I develop my image."

Andy was mired in depression and chained to a floundering business. Yet the predicament of this fledgling entrepreneur was not due to a lack of knowledge of sound business principles. Rather, it was due to emotional insecurity and an inability to project self-confidence. He had the intelligence, skills and drive to become successful. Yet he could not grow his business as fast as he wanted because of his own insecurity.

Whenever the stress at work elevated, Andy became fearful and ceased to execute his business plan. He would invent many reasons for this failure. But the real reason was obvious: stress caused him to freeze.

Andy entered my office complaining of chronic middle back and neck pain. When I palpated the area of his complaint, it was obvious that his problem was more psychological than physical. The muscles were very symmetrically tight across the whole upper back and neck. Whenever there is an injury or a postural problem, muscle spasm is unbalanced. The fact that he had such balanced muscle spasm meant that he was tightening his back and neck muscles subconsciously, probably due to stress.

When Andy and I discussed in more detail what he felt physically and emotionally during these tense sessions, he related that the pain often made it *difficult for him to concentrate. His anxiety would also destroy his ability to focus and memorize important details.*

I told him to use a simple mantra that he could repeat out loud that would bolster his self-confidence. While his business partner was talking, I told him to say, "I understand what you're saying." This phrase had the impact of bolstering his self-confidence and gave him something to say during times of stress.

When he returned the next month, he told me that the program had worked perfectly. He now felt able to control his stress and deal with his partner during these intense meetings.

Unlike our primitive ancestors, we can experience severe stress even though our lives are not threatened. We need strategies to help us relax and remain calm even during an anxiety-producing situation like an intense business meeting.

COMPUTER INCARCERATION

Many of my patients tell me that they feel chained to their workstations. Whether you work for yourself or someone else, sitting in front of the terminal for five to ten hours a day is not uncommon. We forget that this type of behavior is unnatural and unhealthy unless performed with caution. Excessive computer use can have harmful effects upon your eyes, neck, spine and wrists. Prior to the widespread use of computers, typists needed to move to get erasers, paper and carbon. Printing multiple copies of a document required a trip to the mimeograph machine with the complex movements required to perform this task. These days, you spend hours glued to a chair with your eyes fixed on the glare of a computer screen. Printing, faxing and internet surfing are all done at the touch of a button or click of a mouse; we have lost the ability to move.

One of the most important and beneficial changes you can make during your work day is to stand up every half-hour. Even if you continue to look at your screen, standing will relieve a majority of the stress on your back and neck. If you find it difficult to remember to stand up, set a timer, your watch or your computer so that it beeps every thirty minutes to remind you to take a stretch break. Or, stand up every time you print a document.

Also, your posture at your workstation is very important. Notice in Figure 13-1 that the spine is erect, and the legs are at a ninety degree angle to the floor. If you find this position uncomfortable, try sliding

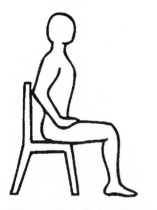

Figure 13-1. Spine Erect; Forearms and Legs Parallel to Floor

your feet a few inches forward on the floor thereby increasing the angle of your legs to greater than ninety degrees.

Ideally, you should be able to change positions often. That is why a sit/stand workstation is ideal. It allows you to go from sitting to standing whenever you feel the need to change positions. If you have a serious lower back problem, try standing at your computer every day for two weeks, and see if it relieves your discomfort. If you have trouble reaching your keyboard or viewing your monitor, stack them on phone books or sturdy boxes.

:60 SECOND MEETING SURVIVAL STRATEGIES

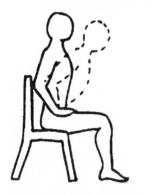

Figure 13-2. Forward-Leaning Position

Long, drawn-out business meetings are often extremely stressful. Long hours in negotiations or planning business strategies can be a cause of both back and neck pain. However, following are a few hints which can make these sessions not only bearable, but a chance to relax and refresh.

It is important to change positions often. After you have spent some time with your back firmly against the back of a chair, try sitting on the edge of your chair with your elbows on the table. Notice in Figure 13-2 how this forward-leaning position can take the pressure off your lower back and place your spine in the neutral position. Try alternating between the standard, upright sitting position and this new posture. You will find that this will significantly relieve back and neck stress.

Once you have achieved both of these positions comfortably, begin to incorporate the quick release techniques for your five stress zones, the belly-chest-exhale breathing techniques and the meditation techniques into your day. Obviously, closing your eyes and meditating for a long period of time during an intense business meeting is impossible. However, there are many ways that you can relax during these stressful events.

During most business meetings, there are moments when the attention shifts to other members of the group. During these periods, close your eyes for approximately one second, inhale, exhale and open your eyes. You will find that this one-second relaxation technique will provide a brief moment of calm during stressful business negotiations. You will find that even this short period of respite will give you the opportunity to become more aware of your posture, breathing and stress level. Use this quick stress release technique whenever you have a limited time during intense business events.

THE FAIL-SAFE STANDING TECHNIQUE

Long hours spent sitting in front of a computer is unhealthy and unnatural. The fail-safe technique for avoiding prolonged periods of sitting involves placing some element of your work into a configuration that forces you to stand up. If you have a bad back or want to avoid getting one, be sure to ask the furniture movers at your company for assistance. Sometimes more than a telephone will need to be moved.

If the telephone is causing a neck problem, you might try purchasing a telephone headset. This will not only free up both hands for writing, but will prevent you from twisting your neck to support the telephone. If you have a back problem as well as a neck problem or find telephone conversations stressful, a wireless telephone headset will allow you to stand up and walk about the room while talking on the telephone. This is a tremendous strategy for relieving back and neck stress and interjecting movement into what is normally a compressive, stressful situation.

MANAGING YOUR FIRST IMPRESSION—
BUSINESS BODY LANGUAGE

Appearance is an important factor in the business world. Where power and pecking order determine business success, managing your impression is a vital part of the business day. Humans are like all other animals and, consciously or unconsciously, view you as friend or foe. In this stressful world of high-powered individuals, your survival will be determined by the impression you make on others. Whether you are dealing with a powerful negotiator on an equal footing or with your boss, there are some secrets to survival.

:60 SECOND COMFORT: SEATED POSITION

If you are concerned about an imbalance in power between you and another individual, always choose the seat that puts you at ease, thereby putting you in a position of power. Decide whether you feel more comfortable sitting with your back against a wall, facing out the window or sitting at the head of the table. Do you prefer the quietest or the noisiest table in a restaurant. Managing your posture and the impression you make requires operating from a position of self-confidence. Take :60 seconds to survey a room and choose the part of a room or an environment which puts you in an advantageous position. If you have not figured out where you feel most comfortable, try sitting in meeting rooms or restaurants by yourself or with friends so you don't feel any pressure and assess where you are most comfortable. Begin to fine-tune this choice into an asset for business success and self-assurance.

:60 SECOND POSTURE AND POWER STRATEGIES

Powerful posture can be attained in either the sitting or standing positions. Remember that you have four :60 second options:

The Mirror

Mirroring the posture of your adversary is a technique designed to make the other person feel more comfortable. The more you look and act like them, the more they will become relaxed and amiable. If they lean back in their chair, you can do the same, while giving them a subtle compliment. Mirroring their posture and telling them how much you like their idea will put them at ease.

The Attack

When you feel the need to make a strong point, to aggressively defend your position or make your adversary feel uncomfortable, try sitting on the edge of your chair, leaning on your elbows and staring into your opponent's eyes. Slightly raise your voice level and enunciate every word clearly. This will add dramatic emphasis to your point. This type of posture is required when you are being attacked and need to defend your position or when you feel the need for some type of verbal victory.

The Loser

You may find it strategically valuable to occasionally give your opponent the impression that they have won. To accomplish this, slump in your chair slightly, look your opponent in the eyes and praise their ideas. Utilizing this type of posture occasionally has great value. For example, if your boss finds fault with something you have done and you desire to display feelings of agreement or remorse, you can use this posture effectively.

The Holding Pattern

There are many times during business meetings that you are uncertain of the shift of power in the negotiations. When this occurs, sit upright, attain a neutral position, relax your stomach muscles and breathe evenly using the belly-chest-exhale breathing technique. By sitting upright, halfway between leaning forward and reclining, you are in a balanced pose, able to be more receptive. Think of this posture as being like an antenna. With your belly soft, while you breathe comfortably, you are better able to receive more accurately the tone and quality of your opponent's discussion.

PUBLIC SPEAKING

The business activity most likely to cause anxiety and perspiration is a required public presentation in front of a group of attentive listeners. Standing in front of a captive audience, with all eyes focused on you, is almost guaranteed to create butterflies in your stomach, not to mention feelings of insecurity. The :60 Second Rejuvenation Strategy can solve this problem.

Your first task is to eliminate, as much as possible, those nervous butterflies commonly associated with public presentation anxiety. The solution is a simple one: use the belly-chest-exhale technique. Breathing slowly, be certain that you inhale the breath into the stomach first, then into the chest, followed by an easy exhale. Be certain that the rate of your breathing is slow and relaxed and that there is a space between your exhalation and your next breath. Because this technique is very subtle and cannot be observed by onlookers, it is an ideal meditation technique to use while speaking. Not only will this technique provoke relaxation, it will also improve your breath control, making the sound quality of your voice far more resonant.

Another very helpful hint is to use the *:60 Second Rejuvenation Strategy's* five stress zones as a focus for relaxation during your presentation. It is quite easy to gently shift your attention up and down through your five stress zones to maintain a sense of calm and intellectual equanimity. While you are talking, move a small part of your attention to each of these areas. After you have noted your feelings in these five primary areas, move your attention back to your breathing. Continue shifting your subconscious attention between your breathing and your five stress zones.

Obviously, you must also follow the basic tenets of proper public speaking, including focusing on one member of the audience at a time, having an organized presentation and using appropriate body language and voice inflection.

:60 SECOND POSTURE THEORY: UNIQUELY STANDING

The *:60 Second Rejuvenation Strategy* teaches standing from the very unique point of view that every individual has a posture that fits his or her unique needs. Here are the techniques that will help you develop your ideal posture:

Feet

First, place your feet approximately hip-width apart. Or, take a few steps, placing your feet the same distance apart as your normal gait. Next, point your feet approximately five degrees outward. If your feet naturally point inward, are parallel or if you feel more comfortable pointing your toes outward, that is how you should place your feet.

Knees

Your knees should be relaxed. To achieve this relaxation, lock your knees into their locked back position, then bend them slightly, as if you are barely squatting. Now find the position in-between those two extremes. This is the neutral knee position; the position in-between being locked back and bent. Continue to move in smaller increments, between this locked position and the bent position, finding the most natural, comfortable place in between. This in-between position should feel like you are on two little ball bearings, balancing in neutral. This is the natural knee position.

Head and Neck

There is a very logical reason for aligning the feet and legs before aligning the head. Your feet are loaded with pressure receptors and nerves that tell your body about your position in space. Also, your feet provide valuable information for the rest of your body about the direction and position in which your head will be most comfortable. If you twist your ankle slightly or step on a stone, the rest of your body will follow. Conversely, your eyes are always scanning your environment, telling your feet that there are steps, a rough patch of gravel or a slope ahead. Thus, the two areas of primary posture control are your feet and your head. That is why we work with the feet first, then the head, followed by the torso.

When you look at your computer, drive your car, speak in front of groups or watch an exciting movie, you are very prone to sticking your neck forward. Because we do this so often, it is important to discover the proper head and neck alignment. First, project your head forward and then pull it back, as if you were a soldier standing at attention. Tuck your chin to your chest so that your head is back in its most retracted position. Now take a deep breath, exhale and relax the neck into its neutral position. The relaxed position that follows head retraction is your ideal head and neck alignment.

Next, turn your head to the left and then to the right, until you feel that your nose is in the middle of your body, facing straight ahead. Later, you might try this in front of a mirror to assess the accuracy of your position.

Shoulders

Children are commonly taught that pulling their shoulders back and standing up straight is the ideal posture. Nothing could be further from the truth. In fact, pulling your shoulders back will cause chronic back and neck tension and pain. To discover your proper shoulder position, pull your shoulders back as if you are squeezing your shoulder blades together. Now relax your shoulders. Next, squeeze your shoulders together in front of you, hollowing out your chest. Now return to the middle position. Perform this exercise a few times until you feel comfortable finding the neutral or natural position in-between the excessively upright posture with the shoulders retracted and the excessively slumped posture with the shoulders forward. This middle position is your natural shoulder alignment.

:60 SECOND RELAXATION TECHNIQUE

Stand comfortably by first placing your feet and knees in the relaxed, neutral positions already described. Next, loosen your neck by tucking your chin and then relaxing it into the neutral position. Move your shoulders forward and back until they feel comfortably in neutral. Now, close your eyes and relax your belly. Breathe using the belly-chest-exhale technique.

The goal of this standing technique is to be able to relax and comfortably enjoy your body while standing, waiting in line or speaking publicly. The next time you are standing, place your body into this neutral posture and then begin breathing with the belly-chest-exhale technique. Closing your eyes for only a few moments is enough to refresh your mind and renew your spirit. If you find this difficult, practice finding the neutral posture in the standing, sitting or supine position. Then try releasing all five stress zones.

:60 SECOND ADVANCED STANDING TECHNIQUE

Now that you have learned the neutral posture while standing and are able to release your five stress zones and breathe comfortably, there is a more advanced technique. It is well known that your standing posture will change according to your mood. As you feel more aggressive, your posture will lunge forward. If you are feeling shy or insecure, you will tend to lean back. To experience this, try this simple technique:

Stand in the neutral position and breathe comfortably. Gently lean forward so your weight shifts to the balls of your feet. Then, shift back to the upright, neutral position. Next, lean back slightly, so you feel the weight shift to your heels. Again, move back to the neutral position. If you close your eyes and allow yourself to explore the forward, neutral and backward positions, you will feel decided differences in your emotional makeup. Whenever you lean forward, your body is poised for action. If you lean back, your body senses a need to retreat.

:60 SECOND BUSINESS BODY LANGUAGE
AND ANXIETY COPING SUMMARY

- At the first indication of rising stress, sit upright, close your eyes for approximately one second, take a deep breath and exhale.
- To bolster your self-confidence and give you something to say during times of stress, use the mantra, "I understand what you're saying."

- Using a timer if necessary to remind you, stand up from your desk or workstation and take a stretch break every thirty minutes.
- Redesign your workspace, relocate your working materials or telephone and consider a headset.
- Choose a seating position where you feel the most comfortable; a position of self-confidence.
- Commit to your memory the four options: The Mirror, The Attack, The Loser and The Holding Pattern.
- Shift your subconscious back and forth between breathing and your five stress zones.
- Determine whether you have created unsuccessful mechanisms for coping, like elevated shoulders, tense facial muscles or continual movement of your hands or fingers, and try to correct them.
- Learn to stand and sit properly—stand your ground.
- Your feet provide valuable information for the rest of your body.
- Learn how to breathe properly and practice the belly-chest-exhale technique—any time, anywhere.
- Make sure you have mastered releasing all five stress zones while standing or sitting.
- Practice the advanced technique in this chapter to experience the decided differences in your emotional makeup as you change positions.

Chapter 14

SEATS—BLESSING OR CURSE

:60 Second Affirmation:
*"On a regular basis,
I change positions and find comfort."*

Mike went to the finest business schools and developed a thriving business leasing high-rise office buildings to Fortune 500 companies. This required long hours of negotiations on the telephone. When he was attacked by a serious bout of lower back pain, he came to me for advice. He told me that when he was working he had absolutely no ability to perceive time passing and was unable to take a break. For Mike, we designed a fail-safe telephone therapy program. I decided to help Mike put movement back in his life by rearranging his office.

Because Mike spent approximately one-third of his time on the telephone, I deduced that these calls would be a great chance for him to stand—as a respite from pounding on his keyboard with his eyes transfixed on his glaring computer screen. I told him to move his telephone off of his desk, onto the top of a series of four-drawer file cabinets behind his desk. Next to the telephone, he placed a writing pad with pens for jotting down notes during serious negotiations. Whenever the phone rang or he desired to make a business call, he was forced to stand up and take a break from the rigors of his sedentary occupation. When Mike returned to my office after trying this new program, he incredulously stated that all of his back pain was gone.

In 1990, a group of researchers in England won the prestigious Volvo Award in Biomechanics and Clinical Science for their work on the relationship of back pain to occupation. They examined the spines of eighty-six cadavers. Having extensive histories of these individuals' work life prior to their deaths, the researchers came to a startling conclusion. They discovered that people who sat for the majority of their work life had degenerated and bulging disks in their lower back. People who were free to sit, stand and walk had healthy spines. There was considerable evidence that long-term chair sitting was actually harmful!

This exciting study helped document that sitting causes the lower back to degenerate. When you sit, the weight of your entire upper body compresses your lower lumbar disks, and because most people slouch when they sit, there are additional stressful forces that make the problem worse. According to this and other studies, standing and walking do not cause the harmful effects that sitting does. There has been a significant increase in back problems over the last century that appears to correlate with the number of hours spent sitting. Although we may believe that sitting is comfortable, it may actually be causing spinal degeneration.

Homo sapiens, 50,000 to 100,000 years ago, were primarily wanderers. They would forage and hunt for food, and only used the most primitive tools and containers. There is no history of chairs being used during this period. Anthropological studies of many nineteenth and twentieth century tribes have shown similar results—primitive people primarily stood or laid down. Occasionally, they would squat or kneel as a break from long hours of standing and walking. However, because they were naked or often scantily clad, they had little desire to sit. After all, the ground was dusty, muddy or crawling with insects. Thus, the healthy lower backs that were discovered in anthropological research of these people may have been due to their lifestyle, since standing and lying down are the ideal positions to prevent spinal degeneration.

During the New Stone Age, around 5,000 to 10,000 B.C., primitive man began to use chairs. Archeological evidence from this era shows benches and ledges designed for sleeping and sitting. In ancient Egypt and Greece, sculptures commonly depict Kings and Pharaohs as sitting upright on elegant thrones. However, at this time, chairs were uncommon among the lower classes—they occasionally used simple stools.

Medieval households rarely used furniture. Small, crude stools and simple benches provided an occasional break from standing and squatting. But by the 1600s to 1700s, padded and more ornate chairs became more common. Because the upper classes had time to socialize, they began to use chairs in place of benches and stools. By the 1800s, simple handmade chairs became quite popular. It was not until the

Industrial Revolution, during the 19th century, when factories began to churn out, on long assembly lines, chairs for office workers.

THE IDEAL CHAIR

There are only two natural positions for the human body, standing and lying down. Any posture must be an outgrowth of one of these two positions. The problem with sitting is that when you elevate your knees to a 90-degree angle to your hips, you round your lower back, causing you to slump. Therefore, the ideal chair will position your knees lower than your pelvis, much like the balance or Balans chair. There are only a few solutions to solve this dilemma:

Sit on a stool

Stools are ideal sitting surfaces around your breakfast nook in the kitchen, at a bar or even in front of your computer workstation. You can raise your computer workstation to standing height, then sit on a stool as a break. Or, purchase an adjustable desk so that you may stand for most of the day, and then lower the desk and sit on your chair to give your legs a well-deserved rest.

Buy an ergonomic chair

The best ergonomic chairs will let you tilt the seat back to mimic a recliner. By tilting the seat back into a reclined position, with your neck supported, you dramatically reduce the stress on your entire spine. Then, when you desire to change positions, you can tilt your seat forward, with your knees below your pelvis, to put your weight on the sits bones and your feet. Both of these positions avoid the pressure on the spine from the typical slumped position caused by the average office chair.

Set up a fail-safe standing arrangement

By organizing your workstation so that about half of your work must be done standing is another strategy. Place your telephone, fax machine, rolodex or printer away from your desk. With these frequently used items out of reach, you will be forced to stand up repeatedly throughout the day.

Buy a recliner

Recliners are the ideal sitting posture for the spine because they support the entire back and neck, without the compressive force of the typical chair. Once you have used a recliner, you may want to sit in nothing else.

Practice lying down

Any chance you get, lie down. Practice being a couch potato at home by stretching out on the couch and reading, rather than sitting in your favorite chair. Practice reclining while watching television, do more work in bed and avoid overstuffed chairs and couches.

DRIVING COMFORT

For most people, driving a car is a common part of everyday life. Commuting to and from work, driving the kids to school and extra-curricular activities, and running errands comprise a large part of many people's daily activities. It is quite common to complete a long period of driving with back or neck soreness. Yet it is possible to drive for long periods of time and avoid these common aches. In fact, it is possible to finish a long drive and feel rested and refreshed. It is even possible to complete a long drive feeling better than before you started!

The problem with driving is a combination of three important factors: First, driving presents all of the problems which we expect from sitting for long periods of time. Secondly, the vibration from the automobile and road surface is very harmful for the back and neck. And lastly, the driving position requires you to use your legs in a very awkward fashion. Because we use the right leg for both the gas pedal as well as the brake, we end up spending most of our driving time in a twisted position.

:60 SECOND CAR SEAT STRATEGY

The simplest and most important way to improve the quality of your driving experience is to recline your car seat. Many people believe that sitting upright, as if they were sitting at a computer or at the dinner table, is appropriate while driving. However, the preferable position for driving should be very similar to the position that you would take while watching a movie, relaxing in your favorite armchair or sitting back in your recliner. Reclining your car seat reduces the weight of your head on your neck and your whole upper body on your lower back. By leaning back in your seat, the force of your weight is pressed into the headrest and seat back rather than into your spine, resulting in a dramatic decrease in pain and fatigue while driving.

Next time you are in your car, plan as if you are going to make your driver's seat into a comfortable chair for eating popcorn and watching a movie before you begin your drive. Bring at least one or two pillows to support your back and neck. Place a back support beneath your lower back and be certain that your neck is in a comfortable position, totally supported by either your headrest or a pillow. You might use throw pillows from your couch, pillows from your bed or an orthopedic support purchased from your local back store.

Adjust the pillows and the seat angle to their optimal position. You need to be upright enough to comfortably reach the steering wheel and see the road. However, with a little bit of practice, you should become extremely comfortable in a more reclined position.

When you are taking long driving trips, you can recline your seat even further to promote comfort. Obviously, if you are driving around town and are forced to look in many directions to watch traffic, you need to elevate your seat back to a higher position. Feel free to elevate and lower your seat back depending upon your activity and driving needs.

Decide what is the ideal seat back position for you based upon the comfort of your back and neck and your ability to see your surroundings clearly. Be certain that your legs are comfortable as well. You might find that moving your seat forward or back will also improve your comfort while driving. When your low back, middle back and neck feel supported and comfortable, you have achieved the optimal driving position. Try driving this way for a period of time. Adjust and modify your seat position until you feel satisfied that you have found the ideal position.

Long, Long Trips

On long trips, it is wise to get out of your car every one to two hours so that you may walk or stretch for :60 seconds. This should be done. While it is important to be comfortable while driving, it is even more important that you take a break from driving if you feel yourself becoming tense or fatigued. Be certain that you take your break at a designated rest stop or a park. This will allow you to safely walk, stretch and loosen up from the stiffening effects of a long drive.

Remember that whatever you do, do the opposite for awhile. If, after driving for a period of time you begin to feel uncomfortable, feel free to modify your driving position. You might find that changing the seat back angle, moving the seat closer or further away from the steering wheel, or modifying your back and neck supports might be helpful. The body does not like to be in any one position for an extended period of time. Feel free to change positions often.

Alternative Car Seat

If you spend a great deal of time driving and find your car seat impossible to make comfortable, you have a number of options. If you can afford it, you may wish to buy a new car with an automatic seat. Automatic seats allow you to easily adjust the seat in almost every direction, with just the touch of a finger. These electric seats are standard equipment on luxury automobiles and are even becoming common on less expensive models.

If you cannot afford to buy a new car, consider buying a new seat. You might purchase a new, replacement seat from your car's manufacturer, or you might consider one of the custom seats which are manufactured by many specialty companies that build quality, long-lasting, comfortable seats. Either way, this is a relatively inexpensive way to get rid of a poorly designed car seat.

If you cannot afford to buy a new seat, but your seat is unusable, consider another alternative. After using pillows for many months, you will be certain where you need increased support in your car seat. Take your car to an upholstery shop and have them rebuild your seat to match the support of the pillows where you find them most comfortable. It is also inexpensive to remove the seat covers and merely add some padding where you feel your seat lacks sufficient support.

If you spend only a few minutes per day in your car, it is unlikely that you will experience any problems as a result of an uncomfortable car seat. However, if you spend more than one or two hours commuting in your car, it is very important that your car seat and driving position be extremely comfortable. By choosing a seat position that supports your natural spinal curves, you are avoiding one of the largest hazards of modern commuting.

:60 SECOND POSITION COMFORT SUMMARY

- Standing and lying down are the ideal positions to prevent spinal degeneration.
- The ideal chair will position your knees lower than your pelvis.
- Practice lying down while watching television, read books in bed and avoid overstuffed couches and chairs.
- Stand up throughout the day to relieve the pressure placed on your back while sitting.
- Before putting your car in gear, decide what the ideal position is for you and recline your car seat in a comfortable position.
- Use comfortable pillows to provide extra support.
- Adjust your steering wheel.
- Walk and stretch for at least :60 seconds every two-hours when on a long trip.
- When you notice yourself tensing up, consciously relax taut muscles.

Chapter 15

THE SPORTING LIFE—
THE REWARDS OF
REASONABLE EXERCISE

:60 Second Affirmation:
*"I exercise to prepare for sports;
I do not do sports for exercise."*

Chuck, a forty-six-year-old emergency room physician, spent all his free time white water rafting, cycling and kayaking in the ocean near his San Francisco home. One day while lifting his kayak, he ruptured a disk in his lower back. He was on the other side of the stethoscope this time, healing from the wounds of his back operation.

Chuck came to my office three months after surgery, a desperate man. Following back surgery, he still had serious left leg pain which radiated into his foot. His lower back was still sore from the surgical incision, and he needed to return to work within the month. This stress was compounded by feelings of withdrawal from cardiovascular exercise. Chuck had been an avid swimmer, jogger, bicyclist, and loved to go kayaking in the San Francisco Bay. But after the surgery, he was still unable to sit for more than fifteen minutes, and he found it impossible to cycle or paddle in his kayak.

My examination determined that Chuck's leg pain was muscular in nature, caused by spasms from irritated nerves in his left leg. Six months of suffering with a lumbar herniated disk had left him with chronically tight leg muscles. I started him on a vigorous leg stretching program, began strengthening his stomach and low back muscles, encouraged him to ice his low back more regularly, *and counseled him to be patient with the healing process. Within a month, much of his left leg pain was gone and the flexibility was returning to his tight leg muscles. The regular icing had reduced his low back discomfort and he was now swimming for fifteen minutes, three times a week. He began to utilize the 5/50 walking program where he was instructed to start walking for five minutes, increasing his distance every five days by fifty percent. Slowly, Chuck was getting back in shape and feeling more comfortable.*

WHAT EXERCISE IS RIGHT FOR YOU?

There are only two kinds of exercise; the exercise you are doing on a regular basis and the exercise you gave up long ago. It is critical to remember that exercise must be fun. You must experience pleasure and enjoyment or you will quickly abandon your regimen.

Mark Twain once said that he had the urge to exercise many times. But if he would just lie on his back and close his eyes, eventually the urge would pass. The question then becomes—what can you do to make exercise enjoyable so that you will desire to perform it on a regular basis? First you must decide if you are a loner or a joiner.

The Loner

Loners enjoy exercise that does not require the participation of other people. Although a loner may be a very sociable person, for many reasons they do not want to depend on others for their physical fitness needs. Loners prefer walking, bicycling, swimming, weight training, yoga, stretching and exercise machines. These types of activities allow them to work out without needing the participation of others.

Another advantage of being a loner is that you can create your own show. Loners often listen to music, read newspapers, books and magazines or watch television while exercising. This "show" may also be an internal one; watching the inner world is also great entertainment for the loner.

The Joiner

The joiner finds solitary exercise to be incredibly boring. They love the thrill of competition and the company of friends and acquaintances as they work out. Joiners love to play golf, tennis, volleyball, basketball, baseball and other competitive sports.

Many people are a combination of these two types. There are many people who go to the gym two or three times a week to keep in shape for their weekend tennis match. Also, many exercise regimens performed by loners may be performed in a group. Joining a swim team, a walking club or a yoga class can provide social activity which gives relief from the repetitious boredom of working out alone.

EXERCISE AND REJUVENATION: THE BALLOON BELLY

I have developed a novel way of ensuring that all of your exercise is performed with your spine in the neutral or natural position. By inhaling fully and holding your breath, you will make it virtually impossible to bend or kink your back into a twisted position. Try the following exercise:

While standing, exhale fully, and notice how easy it is to round your back and bend forward. Then try bending to the side. Now take a very deep breath down into your belly and hold it. This *balloon belly technique* will make it almost impossible for you to round your back while bending forward or to the side. You will find that the balloon belly will keep your spine in a stable position. Any time you are performing heavy physical labor, lifting a heavy box or trying a new exercise, use the balloon belly technique to prevent the dangers of a contorted spine.

For example, if you are a golfer, perform a few practice swings with the balloon belly. You will find that every sport will be performed more safely with your spine in the neutral position. The balloon belly will ensure that you do not round your back, preventing the possibility of spinal injury. Although this technique is often used by professional athletes, it works just as well for less active people.

HUFF AND PUFF,
:60 SECOND STRETCH AND STRENGTHEN

The ideal exercise program involves three basic elements:

1. *Huff and puff:* Aerobic exercise to strengthen the heart and lungs.
2. *Stretching:* Flexibility exercises to maintain comfort and good range of motion.
3. *Strengthening:* Muscle strength for stability and to prevent osteoporosis.

The ideal exercise program should involve these three elements. Ideally you should perform some stretching to ensure flexibility and muscular comfort. Yoga, stretching programs and the *:60 Second Rejuvenation Strategy* exercises are good examples of what can be done to improve flexibility.

Strengthening exercises are best performed using free weights or weight machines. However, there are many new cardiovascular machines, such as the cross-country ski machine, which require you to perform aerobic functions and strengthen your upper, as well as your lower body. Aerobic exercise requires you to elevate your heart rate for at least fifteen to thirty minutes. Walking, jogging, bicycling and swimming are excellent examples of safe cardiovascular exercise.

EXERCISE USING THE :60 SECOND REJUVENATION STRATEGY

Remember to use the balloon belly when you return to your favorite exercise. It will easily teach you how even stressful games such as golf, tennis, weightlifting and basketball can be enjoyed with your spine in the natural, neutral position.

Walking

Walking is an ideal exercise. It is safe, relaxing, strengthens the heart and lungs and reduces the risk of osteoporosis. For variety, switch between walking in your neighborhood, using a treadmill or taking a long hike at the beach or in the mountains. If you like to be entertained, think about getting audio tapes or CDs containing music or your favorite books on tape.

Swimming

Swimming is an ideal exercise because your body is supported by the water, reducing the likelihood of the damaging effects of compression and impact. Here are a few hints:

1. Use a snorkel. It will reduce your need to turn your head while doing the crawl.
2. Vary your strokes using the crawl, breast stroke, side stroke and back stroke, so that you use all of your muscles equally.
3. Use swim fins. They will reduce the stress on your shoulders and provide more exercise for your legs.

Weight Training

Weight machines are safer than free weights because you do not need to lift the weights off of a rack or stabilize them. However, light hand and ankle weights are an excellent addition to any exercise program.

Make sure that you always work all sides of a muscle. For example, when strengthening the legs, make sure you strengthen the front, back, inside and outside of your leg muscles to maintain proper muscular balance and healthy posture.

If you have not used weight machines or free weights before, it is very important to have a qualified trainer show you the proper way to use them the first time to avoid injury. Most gyms and health clubs provide this service for free (included in your membership fee).

Yoga

Yoga is an ideal exercise because it provides both balance and flexibility. Always perform yoga slowly and cautiously. Be careful of overstretching. Do not perform any exercises, such as standing on your head, performing aggressive twists or deep forward bends unless you are an advanced student. There are many fine books on yoga and stretching to help you develop a safe and effective practice.

Competitive Sports

Golf, tennis, volleyball, basketball, baseball and other competitive sports can easily result in sudden injury. Always remember to try the balloon belly technique before or after a game to make sure that you are following the tenets of the *:60 Second Rejuvenation Strategy*. No matter how much you want to win, try to remember to use natural posture and not dive, twist or jump in a reckless haphazard fashion. Even professional athletes with big money riding on every game know that one wrong move could sideline them for a season. Sports are pleasurable activities but can involve risk. Always try to exercise two days for every day playing sports. Stretching, strengthening and aerobic exercise will prepare you for your competitive games.

:60 SECOND SPORTS PREPARATION SUMMARY

- Determine if you are a loner or a joiner or perhaps a combination of the two.
- Remember, you will only continue to exercise if it is enjoyable.
- Try the balloon belly technique whenever you exercise or perform a sports activity.
- Huffing and puffing, stretching and strengthening are the three basic elements for ideal exercise.
- Use exercise to prepare for sports; don't do sports for exercise.

Chapter 16

PERFORMING AND ENJOYING THE ARTS

:60 Second Affirmation:
"Whatever I do, I do the opposite for a while
and stay within the golden zone."

A successful San Francisco artist, Anita had developed a wide following in the San Francisco Bay area for her large murals and complex landscapes. The sudden onset of shoulder and forearm pain forced her to stop painting. Because her career and productivity were at risk, she consulted me for help with her disabling condition—tendonitis. Anita's career was threatened by a common but extremely painful condition produced by overuse of forearm or wrist muscles.

I explained to Anita that the tendonitis which caused the severe pain in her right shoulder, arm and hand could be easily eliminated with proper posture and exercise. I helped her understand that the way she positioned her easel was the probable cause of her injury and that repetitive use of her arm in the incorrect position caused her muscles to become inflamed. This inflammation would heal with time but would form microscopic amounts of scar tissue. This scar tissue could eventually form around the muscles and tendons, creating a chronic condition. This condition is also seen often in cashiers and secretaries who work for long hours with their wrists held in an improper position.

I asked Anita to show me exactly how she painted in her studio. As I watched her perform large, imaginary brushstrokes, I saw that she positioned her large canvasses either on the floor or on a high easel. I noticed that she was either bending over on the floor in a cramped position or having to reach above the natural limitations of her petite posture. I showed her the normal reach for someone her size–the area from her eyes to her waist. I explained that anything above or below that was outside the golden zone, which is the area easily reached with normal arm movements and told her that we would need to redesign her body mechanics.

When she returned the following week, she told me that most of her pain was gone. She realized that she needed to modify her easel; her large canvasses were either too high or too low. She began working with three easels of different heights, which allowed her to comfortably reach all parts of her canvas without painful straining.

Whether you are enjoying art as a spectator or a performer, the same principles apply–relieve the stress from your five stress zones, breathe using the belly-chest-exhale technique and keep your body in its neutral position.

FILM, MUSIC AND THE THEATER

Enjoying a good movie or your favorite dance or musical performance can be enjoyable or painful. It is common to squirm during the final movements of a symphony or ache after long periods of time in uncomfortable movie theater seats. However, it is possible to learn how to sit during a concert, theater or dance performance without fleeing before intermission.

Although many theaters now provide comfortable seating, the quality of seating is still a gamble. The biggest problem with most seats is that they are set at a rigid angle, which often causes you to slump, putting stress on your lower neck and back. If you have a low back support which you use in your chair or car, bring it into the theater and see if this helps.

Another suggestion is to alternate between sitting against the seat back and moving your buttocks a few inches forward in the seat. Filling in this space with a pillow or backrest can provide a welcomed relief from sitting upright. Many back and travel stores sell inflatable pillows, which you can inflate or deflate, allowing you to change positions to reduce the stress on your lumbar spine.

If using a backrest or changing positions are not sufficient in variety to eliminate your back or neck pain, try choosing an aisle seat so that you may get up every half-hour to stretch your back and legs.

Almost all theaters and concert halls now have seating for persons with disabilities, as well as places to stand when the theater is overflowing with patrons. When ordering tickets, inquire about purchasing a seat where you are able to conveniently stand without interrupting the performance. Most theaters have had this request before, and they are happy to comply with your need for a comfortable seat. Or, if the theater is on a first-come, first-serve basis, get to the theater early and find an aisle seat, in the back row, where you can quietly and unobtrusively get up out of your seat to relieve stress on your back or neck.

READING

Delving into a good book, magazine or newspaper can be a wonderful way to relax. However, curling up on an overstuffed couch can make it difficult to uncurl. Remember that even the simple act of reading is more enjoyable when you utilize the :60 Second Rejuvenation Strategy. Many overstuffed couches are actually very poorly designed—they emphasize home decor rather than true comfort and do not support the natural curves of your back.

The ideal way to read is in a recliner, with your book propped up near eye-level. If you do not have a recliner, think about purchasing one. They are often sold at garage sales for $100 or less or may be purchased from high-end back and chair stores for $1,000 to $2,000. Either way, the same principle applies. If you are in a semi-reclined position and place your reading material at a more natural height, you will take the pressure off of your spine and neck.

If you have no recliner, try reading while lying flat on your back, with your head slightly elevated, and a pillow under your arms and hands to elevate your reading material up to eye-level. Then, as a break from reclining, sit at a table with your book propped up on a reading stand or some object that allows you to angle the book up off of the table or desk. This will prevent you from having to bend your neck over to look at your book or newspaper. Alternatively, standing for short periods of time while reading is another choice.

One very important rule for emotional and physical well-being is to avoid repetitive motions. I teach my patients the mantra, *Whatever you do, do the opposite for a while.* Many of them, during a two- to three-hour reading session, will alternate half-hour segments of lying down, sitting and standing. They find that this virtually eliminates any stress on their back or neck, aids in proper breathing and allows them to vary the muscles which are being used.

ARTISTIC EXPRESSION

Artistic expression of a new kind requires a relaxed, aligned body with proper breathing. It is impossible to tap the deep roots of your creative soul while your breath is labored or your neck is contorted in an unbalanced position. Professional dancers are aware of these facts and constantly work on proper body alignment to promote grace and proper breathing.

Whether you are taking your first lambada or ballroom dancing lesson or struggling through an aerobics class, dancing can be a joy or a source of tremendous frustration. Being out of step with the music or forgetting the routine can cause stress and anxiety. These problems are easily eliminated by using the *:60 Second Rejuvenation Strategy*.

If you are already worried about your next dance or aerobics class, just practice one aspect of the *:60 Second Rejuvenation Strategy* at a time. For example, for the first class or lesson, only pay attention to your breathing and be certain that you are breathing using the belly-chest-exhale technique. You will find that proper, fluid breathing will aid in your natural body alignment and will promote relaxation. During the next class, focus on your five stress zones, making certain that they are all in the relaxed and open position. Once you have worked on proper breathing and have eliminated muscle tension, focus on maintaining a neutral posture. Virtually all dance techniques teach these principles of proper breathing, relaxation and body alignment.

I have treated many musicians, painters, dancers and actors. They have all told me that when they are performing at their highest level, their body is in perfect alignment, their breathing is easy and their muscles feel fluid and relaxed. Musicians and writers find these principles help them reduce creative blocks. They talk about increased energy flow through proper breathing, relaxation and body alignment.

Playing a musical instrument can be a joy when you realize that you need not play in a contorted, twisted position. If you are struggling with any type of creative expression, do not try to change everything at once. Continue to use the body as you have in the past. Each day that you practice, focus on one element of the *:60 Second Rejuvenation Strategy*, striving for more relaxation, a more neutral posture and more relaxed breathing. Even violinists, with chronic cricks in their necks, have learned to elevate their chin just a few millimeters, taking stress off important nerves in the neck and back.

:60 SECOND PERFORMANCE AND SPECTATOR COMFORT SUMMARY

- Redesign body mechanics so you stay within the *golden zone*.
- Practice relieving stress from your five stress zones, breathe using the belly-chest-exhale technique and keep your body in its neutral position.
- Bring low back support to seated events or choose a seat on an aisle or where you are able to alternate standing and sitting.
- When reading, alternate between a reclined position and a seated position, as well as standing.
- Remember the mantra, "Whatever you do, do the opposite for a while and stay within the golden zone."

Chapter 17

CREATING SEXUAL PLEASURE—
THE POSTURE/PLEASURE CONNECTION

:60 Second Affirmation:
"Loving myself, I open to others."

A fifty-four-year-old engineer and physicist, Sam was selected as the director of research at a respected university think tank. Along with travel, consulting with major universities and foreign capitals, Sam had a busy, intense family life. This meticulously detailed and planned life was rudely interrupted by a routine medical exam, confirming that he had prostate cancer. Although he dealt well with the surgery, he was depressed by the resulting impotence caused by the procedure. Sex had become a stressful and humiliating experience for him.

Sexual intercourse, in our society, is almost entirely focused on genital pleasure. There is very little mention of the slow, gentle intimacy that characterizes healthy, loving sexual relationships. This focus on the genitals, rather than emotions or bodily sensations, can be disastrous. Sam was forced to confront these issues.

Sam no longer derived pleasure from sexual intercourse with his loving wife. I helped Sam realize that he could receive pleasure without an erection, and that he could feel excitement in other parts of his body. Sam transformed his sensual orientation from a focus on orgasm as a final goal to a higher level of pleasure and emotional intimacy. He described his new lovemaking style as touching, nurturing and foreplay rather than excitement, contact and orgasm. His real breakthrough came when he discovered a new kind of orgasm. Long, sensual lovemaking sessions without orgasm produced what he described as emotional bubbles.

After extensive lovemaking, he would experience what he described as carbonation bubbling throughout his body. He had learned to experience a deeper and subtler form of sexual pleasure.

SEX: SAFETY, SENSUALITY, SENSITIVITY AND SIN

Hollywood portrays flawless, unblemished sexual encounters. The silver screen does not often portray the trauma of failed orgasm, impotence, performance anxiety or emotionally detached lovemaking. Consequently, we are commonly disappointed when our sexual encounters do not match the wild, but perfect, passion of our movie heartthrobs and idols. These glorious but sterile portrayals of sexuality are almost impossible to achieve. Sex and love almost always result in some disappointment and heartache.

We need to develop a new form of sexuality that emphasizes a more primitive sensitivity and avoids the neurotic focus upon performance and perfection.

PROCREATION VS. RECREATION

Some feel that sex is only for making babies, some characterize sex as an almost religious or mystical activity and others see it as a natural part of an intimate connection with a partner. The latter view best demonstrates healthy sexuality. Healthy, loving relationships focus on emotional and physical intimacy that naturally leads to sensuality. Sexuality must be an outgrowth of physical and emotional pleasure.

LOVE VS. LUST

The ideal sex life is a natural outgrowth of a healthy body and sane attitudes. Scientific surveys commonly report that loving, married couples often achieve very satisfying sex lives. It is quite difficult to have a long-term and vibrant sexual life when you are regularly on the prowl for a new partner. A loving partner can tenderly accept our weaknesses and allow us to express deep affection. Yet many of us do not have a partner for sharing sexual experiences. That poses an obvious dilemma.

MARRIAGE, MONOGAMY AND MASTURBATION

If you do not have a healthy, monogamous marriage, you only have a few choices. You can be celibate, you can masturbate or you can have a sexual affair. Obviously, celibacy is the safest choice. Abstaining from any sexual activity prevents the possibility of sexual transmitted diseases, while protecting you from the disappointment inherent in affairs and one-night stands. Yet avoiding all sexual contact can be frustrating and lonely.

THE SENSIBLE, SENSUAL SOLUTION

Because the *:60 Second Rejuvenation Strategy* always focuses on using natural solutions based upon biology and evolution, it discourages the artificial. Thus, titillating movies and pornography conflict with the Rejuvenation Strategy. If you are single, you can still explore your sexuality. But increased sexual awareness or masturbation should come from natural healthy emotion and should not be artificially stimulated.

:60 SECOND SEXUAL AWARENESS EXERCISES

The following exercises are designed to teach you to increase your level of body awareness. The *:60 Second Rejuvenation Strategy* teaches that healthy body awareness naturally produces sensuality, creating the opportunity for wholesome sexual expression. These exercises can improve your body awareness and help you discover comfortable sexual positions that provoke the highest level of sensual feelings.

All of the exercises are designed to be performed alone and in the privacy of your own home. Your bed is an ideal surface to lie on, but a mat or a carpeted floor will also work.

NOTE: Do not perform any of the following exercises if they provoke pain.

The Pelvic Rock

Lie on your back with your knees up and your feet flat on the floor. Gently flatten your lower back as your genitals rise slightly. If you have trouble with these movements, place both hands beneath the arch in your lower back and practice pressing your lower back down into your hands and then relaxing back to neutral. Try performing this exercise, breathing through your nose, with your mouth closed. You will find that the movement is very satisfying and calming when performed this way. It is most natural to inhale as your back arches upward and to exhale as your back flattens. Some people call this exercise the *pelvic rock* as it is an important part of any back care program.

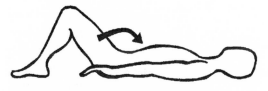

Figure 17-1. The Pelvic Rock

If you desire more sensual stimulation, try breathing through your mouth. Try performing this exercise instead of masturbating. The movements and breathing can be quite satisfying, even without an orgasm. Try exhaling with a sound as your genitals gently rise from the bed and your back flattens. This will provoke even more emotional release and will provide increased body awareness.

The Cobra

In yoga, the *cobra* is an important exercise to relax the lower back and improve posture. Do not perform this exercise or any of the other exercises in the book if they provoke pain.

Lie flat on your stomach while propping yourself up on your elbows. Allow your lower back to gently stretch downward until you feel comfortable in this position. First, gently breathe in and out through your nose, experiencing the relaxation of this position. If you desire more stimulation, breathe through your mouth. The cobra exercise becomes more sexual if you use your arm and chest muscles to gently lift your pelvis off the bed. In this position, you can very gently perform the pelvic rock exercise to provoke deeper, sensual feelings.

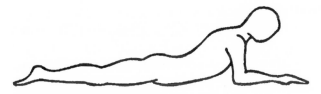

Figure 17-2. The Cobra

The Bridge

Lie on your back in the same position which you utilized for the pelvic rock. Lift your buttocks so that your pelvis is comfortably suspended off the ground. You may lift or lower your pelvis to achieve maximum comfort. In this position, gently breathe, first through your nose and then

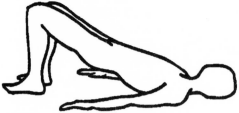

through your mouth, adding sounds if they feel comfortable. This strengthens the lower back and pelvis and can deepen your ability to perceive sensual pleasure.

Figure 17-3. The Bridge

Kegel

A classic exercise for strengthening your sexual and urinary systems is called the *Kegel*. Tighten the muscles at the base of your pelvis as if you are trying to stop the flow of urine. Hold for ten seconds and release. You can practice Kegels any time, sitting or standing, but they are especially powerful when performed along with the pelvic rock, cobra and bridge exercises.

SEXUAL POSTURE

Sexual intercourse is most enjoyable when you know what you want. You must be aware of what positions or postures are right for you. Most of the time, you will either be on your back or on your stomach. Although there are other interesting and erotic positions that you may use, you will probably find yourself returning to these two basic postures. There are four common sexual positions.

The Missionary Position

Every culture has fads and fantasies about the best position to use when making love. However, the missionary position with the man or woman on top, is extremely popular because it is mutually satisfying. This position allows a tremendous amount of freedom of movement. This freedom allows each partner to move in ways that are mutually satisfying. From this position it is possible to move onto the side, change who is on top or bottom or rise to the standing position. Varying positions can add interest and excitement.

The decision as to who is on top is quite flexible. Often a partner with back pain will choose to be on the bottom. The missionary position is ideal because it allows either partner to be on the top or bottom and allows face-to-face contact. Other positions, although quite erotic, do not offer this type of intimacy.

Birds Do It, Bees Do It

In the animal kingdom, it is quite common for the female to stand squarely on all four legs while the male enters from the rear. In humans, the woman is typically on her hands and knees, while her partner kneels behind her, gently entering her vagina with his pelvis up against her buttocks. This can also be an extremely satisfying and comfortable position, although it lacks the intimacy of face-to-face contact. This is an excellent position for a woman with back pain because it allows her to be stable, comfortable and free from pressure on her spine. Although this posture is quite comfortable for men and women, it lacks the direct pressure on the clitoris, which is so satisfying in the missionary position. However, with a bit of ingenuity, the man or woman can stimulate the clitoris and resolve this problem. Another variation on this position is for the woman to lie on her stomach, with the man lying face down on her back, also entering from the rear.

Side Lying

Many couples find it quite comfortable for both partners to lie on their side. Although this provides face-to-face contact, it does not allow for free and balanced motion of the pelvis. Unless you are careful, it can cause you to twist and put unnecessary strain upon your spine. However, you might try these positions with one partner half on their back, with support from behind by pillows. The other partner can be on top, missionary style, with one side of their body on the bed. This position is ideal for a partner with back pain who is most comfortable lying on one side.

Up, Up and Away

Many couples find it quite satisfying for both of them to stand or to kneel, facing each other. The problem is obvious. Although this provides excellent face-to-face contact and intimacy, any difference in heights will be magnified dramatically. If this is a comfortable position for lovemaking, but your heights make it ungainly, try having one partner stand or kneel on two phone books of equal height. Place one book under each foot or knee or use some other very stable platform. This position may be more comfortable if one partner is up against the wall in a braced, stable position.

TO THINE OWN SELF BE TRUE

The basis of a healthy sexual relationship must include a high level of body awareness. Before trying to master or experiment with the positions which have been mentioned, spend most of your time understanding your own true needs. It is most important to find out which postural positions feel comfortable for you before engaging in lovemaking.

While human beings have been enjoying sex for thousands of years, only recently have we been bombarded with technical information describing both deadly diseases and the perfect romance possible from intercourse. Remember that a healthy sensual relationship should be based on deep feelings of love with a high level of body awareness. Also, remember that loving yourself is a prerequisite for loving others.

:60 SECOND SEXUAL PLEASURE ENHANCEMENT SUMMARY

- Healthy, loving sexual relationships focus on emotional and physical intimacy that naturally leads to sensuality.
- The basis of a healthy sexual relationship must include a high level of body awareness.
- The :60 Second Rejuvenation Strategy teaches that improved body awareness naturally produces sensuality, creating the opportunity for wholesome sexual expression.
- Sexual relations are most enjoyable when you know what you want.
- Remember that loving yourself is a prerequisite for loving others.

Chapter 18

REMEMBERING AND
ACHIEVING YOUR GOALS

:60 Second Affirmation:
"I look inside, I stay in touch with my inner self."

Anna, an accomplished computer programmer from Taiwan, was struggling to balance the demands of married life, two children and sixty-hour work weeks at a booming high-tech company. Her husband, tired of not seeing his wife, complained that he felt like a single parent. A few months later, when Anna continued her hectic pace, she saw her family less and less. Finally, her husband filed for divorce.

Anna's marital upheaval lead her to immerse herself even more in her work. And, in spite of chronic back and leg pain, she would forget to take stretch breaks. When she came home in the evenings she would be too exhausted to stretch or exercise and usually would sit and watch television or go right to bed.

The stress of her harried lifestyle and divorce, juxtaposed with her chronic lower back pain and sciatica, created feelings of depression and panic. She finally realized she had to make a change. Anna considered seeing a psychiatrist as well as an orthopedic surgeon or a chiropractor. She decided to come to my office.

In our first interview, I got a sense of what Anna was going through. She tearfully told me of her divorce. She felt betrayed by her husband's lack of support and was angry at him for breaking up their marriage and family. And, despite the financial success she was experiencing, she resented her job as well for its role in her failed marriage. I recommended that she seek therapy or psychological counseling. I also took the opportunity to explain the healthy triangle, which involves a balance of love, work and spirituality. I asked her to reflect on her life and how the healthy triangle applied to her. We discussed how the focus on her work caused an imbalance in her life, which ultimately lead to many of her problems. I wanted her to see that there were many factors that lead to her feelings of resentment and despair, but that she could not continue to blame others; she had to look to herself for answers and for change. She told me she was eager to change. I referred her to a psychologist for help with her emotional pain and then she and I began working on her physical pain.

She had already seen a physical therapist who had given her a list of many exercises. However, she quickly abandoned her program because the regimen required forty-five minutes to perform. Although she came to me ready to change her ways, I realized that it would be best for her to start with an exercise and stretching program that was easily remembered and could be quickly performed while she was at her office. First, I taught her about the "anchor" memory aid.

Since Anna always wore a watch on her left wrist, I suggested she wear it on her right wrist for the next few weeks. As she moved her watch from her left wrist to her right, I could see her struggling with the uncomfortable notion. I told her that the point of the exercise was to create a strange sensation that would act as a reminder that she should stand up from her computer at least every thirty minutes. Each time she noticed the strange sensation of her watch on her right wrist, she was to look at it and assess how long she had been sitting. If it had been more than thirty minutes, she should get up, walk around and perform a few stretching exercises. I also suggested that if she began to get used to having the watch on her right wrist, she should move it back to her left wrist to continue to provide the strange sensation that would be her reminder. Within a few weeks, Anna reported that the anchor memory aid had worked: she was remembering to get up and stretch and her back pain was greatly alleviated.

THE HEALTHY TRIANGLE

In geometry, the triangle is an exceedingly stable structure, composed of three angles and three lines—a strong enough shape to provide the foundation for many buildings and bridges. In life, the healthy triangle is three elements that support a healthy existence: love, work and spirituality.

Love

Love involves all elements of emotional connection with people. Husbands, wives, friends, lovers and children provide richness and meaning to life. Without love, life is like dry, barren and parched earth.

Work

Although most people earn a living through toil of some kind, the most stimulating work involves contributing in some way to society or family as well as self-fulfillment.

Spirituality

It is helpful to feel a connectedness to a higher power or a spiritual belief. Treating the body as a temple can lead to emotional and spiritual health. This can give rise to a healthy lifestyle.

The healthy triangle is not only made up of these three elements, but each element depends on the other; if one element is lacking, it causes the others to be diminished. For example, it is quite rare to have a commitment to spirituality and self-improvement without meaningful relationships and rewarding work. If each element is nurtured and cultivated, all three will flourish and improve the quality of your life.

THREE WAYS TO MAKE :60 SECOND TECHNIQUES WORK

The :60 Second Anchor Memory Aid

An anchor prevents a ship from drifting off at sea. An anchor memory aid is designed to keep you focused on a program and not allow you to drift away from this focus. It can be any device or aid that keeps you focused on any activity you tend to forget or get distracted from doing.

There are many other ways to create anchors. Some people like to use a timer on a watch or clock that will beep at intervals. Teenagers often draw pictures or write notes on their hands with a pen. For women, a new bracelet could perform the same function. Many people find that putting their ring on a different finger is also quite effective. Or, placing a sticker on your computer screen will also work. Anything that will regularly get your attention and remind you to perform a task will be effective.

The 5/50 Rule

The 5/50 rule means that you should start any new program for five minutes or perform five repetitions. Do this for a minimum of five days. For example, if you want to walk a half-hour every day, start with five minutes. Walk for five minutes every day for five days. If you are successful with this program, then walk for seven and a half minutes, a fifty percent increase. After five more days, increase your walking time again by fifty percent, and so on. This 5/50 rule prevents you from increasing any program so rapidly that you cause injury or push yourself too strenuously and then become discouraged.

Anchor Memory Aid in Diet And Weight Loss

Losing weight is one of life's most difficult tasks. Yet it becomes much easier when you incorporate the elements of our unique anchor memory aid. In this case, we will use a slight twist with our technique. This time we will focus on one food. Choose only one food as your anchor. You should choose the food in your diet which is highest in fat or sugar or a food that you compulsively eat. Foods such as ice cream, candy bars, fatty meats, donuts, etc., should be your first choice. Once you have chosen this food, you may either eliminate the food entirely or substitute a healthier alternative.

You must make the decision that you are not going to eat that particular food ever again. Although this sounds quite extreme, it is the same technique used by addicts to give up cigarettes, alcohol and drugs. They find it is easier to give up the drug entirely than to sample it once in a while.

If you are overweight, try taking the one worst food in your diet that you compulsively eat and give it up. If you love to eat donuts, for example, try substituting muffins, bagels or croissants. However, the key to focusing on this one food is to never eat this food again, without trying to eliminate any other food for a minimum of three to six months. Give yourself time to change your lifestyle. You may have some difficulty or you may find yourself learning that you have significantly more will power than you originally thought.

If you could eliminate only the one worst food in your diet and perform this exercise every six months, you will be able to eliminate the two worst foods from your diet forever. Anyone who eliminates the two fattiest, most sugar-laden foods from their diet will lose weight. Eventually, you will find yourself eating healthier foods such as fruits, vegetables and lean meats.

Also important to note is that it is easier to remember to not eat one food for a few months than it is to think about slight restrictions on your entire diet. Anchoring on this one food allows you to eat all the good foods that you want. Also, all low-fat foods should be eaten in abundance if you are trying to eliminate your "nemesis" food.

:60 SECOND GOAL TIPS SUMMARY

- Remember that work, love and spiritual growth—the three aspects of The Healthy Triangle—are the foundation of a healthy life.
- Use the Anchor Memory Aid to help you remember to perform an exercise.
- Use a ring, watch, bracelet or some other device to remind you to perform an exercise.
- Always follow the 5/50 rule: increase or decrease any program by only fifty percent and stick to it for at least five days.
- The next time you try to diet, just eliminate the one food highest in fat or calories and work with this one food for a minimum of three to six months.
- Take small steps to achieve your goals.

PART 4

INCREASING WELLNESS
AND LONGEVITY

Chapter 19

MUSCLES—PAIN AND PLEASURE

:60 Second Affirmation:
"Taking care of myself frees me from pain."

Paula was experiencing muscular pain and dizzy spells. Neurologists, orthopedists, ear specialists, chiropractors, physical therapists, massage therapists and acupuncturists had no idea what was causing her pain or dizziness. One slight move of the head, an incorrect movement in bed or craning her neck while driving her car would result in shooting pain.

During our first session, I gently loosened the muscles and bones in Paula's lower and middle back. I was wary of treating her neck, because she informed me that any movement of her neck could send her spinning off balance. Since her orthopedic and neurologic exams yielded no abnormal findings, I proceeded to gently massage her tight neck muscles. My first contact with the lateral muscles of her neck caused her to grab my hand forcefully, explaining that my touch had provoked the dreaded outcome. I waited for her dizziness to pass and began to review what I could have done to provoke such a response.

Using only my fingertips, I began examining the skin, then the superficial muscles near the sensitive area. I discovered a tiny line, about 1-1/2 inches long and 1/4-inch wide, which was unusually sensitive. All the other skin and muscles in the area appeared to be normal, but this area felt slightly different. She told me that the area felt tender and electric. I decided to use gentler pressure but go deeper.

The area was in the approximate location of a major nerve in the neck. I discovered that the skin over that area and the muscles beneath it did not want to stretch when my fingers attempted to gently pry them apart. Over time, I continued to work with her neck, stretching the tight muscles over the sensitive area; trying to stretch what felt like a taut rubber band beneath the surface of her skin. At the end of this session, she told me that her experience felt like I was irritating a small electric wire embedded in her muscles. I reasoned that the only logical possibility could be that a nerve in her neck had somehow been damaged or had actually grown in an abnormal fashion, embedding itself in her neck muscles. I asked her to stretch her neck muscles in a very specific way, hoping to lengthen what I now thought was a tiny nerve being strangled.

When Paula returned for her third session, she said her neck felt significantly better. I discovered that she had not been taught how to prevent pain and also did not understand how to treat herself when the pain reached frightening levels. I started her on a program of intensive education which resulted in a pain-free back for the first time in years. As future sessions progressed, using gentle cranial mobilizations, deep massage therapy and stretching exercises, we eventually got rid of a majority of the pain, and the frightening sensitivity she had been experiencing was relieved.

MUSCLE MEMORY

Tissue heals, but muscle remembers. Embedded in each muscle are tiny structures called *muscle spindles* and *golgi tendon organs*. Functioning as *rheostats*, these structures are similar to thermostats which can be set to maintain a specific level of heating or cooling. Once these tiny spindles and organs have learned to shorten, they know nothing else.

Interlaced throughout your muscles are millions of nerves which connect to your spinal cord and brain. Since there is no separation between the human brain and these tiny nerves, they serve as a continuous, vibrant feedback system. The brain contains memory which influences muscle function, but memory is contained in muscles as well. Researchers have found that many simple reflexes occur between the spinal cord and this web of nerves which runs throughout the muscles in the body. Muscles, when touched or stretched, may produce profound and graphic memories which can lie dormant until provoked. What is not fully understood is the physiological or hormonal processes which underlie muscle memory.

One aspect of the *:60 Second Rejuvenation Strategy* involves releasing tiny knots in muscles called *trigger* or *tender* points. As these points melt from sustained pressure and massage, many beneficial results can be attained. A well-trained massage therapist, physical therapist or chiropractor can provide deep massage therapy to loosen these tight, stiff muscular points. However, the :60 *Second Rejuvenation Strategy* is based upon what you can do for yourself in a minute or less.

MANAGING YOUR PAIN

The following are the most important tips for managing pain. These hints have helped thousands of my patients lessen pain or become pain-free.

COLD THERAPY

Ice is the ideal therapy for any acute injury. This means that any new injury should be treated first with ice, before ever considering heat. Cold, as a therapy, reduces inflammation and relieves pain almost instantly. However, it must be utilized properly to be safe and effective.

Put the cold pack on the area of pain for five to fifteen minutes, every two hours during the period of greatest pain. As the pain decreases, you may use this cold therapy less frequently. Decrease to every few hours and then a few times per day until the pain is gone.

Whenever you are using an ice pack, always wrap a paper towel or thin kitchen dishtowel around the outside of the pack. This will avoid freezing the surface of your skin and causing more inflammation. As it begins to warm up, the ice pack may lose some of its effectiveness. At this point, you might want to take off the towel to provide a colder surface.

Making Your Own Ice Pack

Inexpensive, effective ice packs are available in your local pharmacy or drug store. If you injure yourself but do not have an ice pack around, you can improvise one easily. A bag of frozen peas or corn works well as an ice pack because it is quite pliable and conforms to the shape of your body.

You can also make a slushy ice pack by mixing three cups of water with one cup of rubbing alcohol. Pour this mixture into a zip-lock bag until it is approximately half full. Place a second zip-lock bag around the outside. Then, put this mixture in the freezer and you will soon have a cold, flexible ice pack. You may also take ice cubes or crushed ice and put them into a plastic or zip-lock bag. Always put a second bag around the outside to prevent leakage as the ice cubes melt. Other suggestions include putting a damp towel in the freezer or using an ice cube to massage the sore area. Always use ice on an acute or new injury. Heat is only for old, chronic or mild problems.

HEAT

A hot tub, sauna or down comforter are soothing therapies for pain and distress. Heat is the ideal therapy for all types of very mild aches and pains. Yet it should never be used when you have acute or serious pain. Since heat increases the blood supply to the area, it should never be used when there is acute or serious inflammation.

However, if you are merely feeling sore and stiff, try warming the area with a heating pad, taking a hot bath, enjoying a sauna or using a hot water bottle. After five to ten minutes of warmth, try some very gentle stretching. You might find that this stretching will be easier and more effective after warming the area. This occurs because warmth relaxes muscles and allows them to stretch more easily.

REST

Years ago, before the age of super drugs and wonder cures, doctors and healers prescribed rest as a primary therapy. This therapy has been forgotten as we have become more dependent on pharmaceutical solutions and less willing to take time off from our busy schedules. We anguish over missed days from work and an apparently infinite number of errands and chores, striving for financial success. Yet relaxation is far better than medication for healing many of life's ailments. Years ago, it was popular for doctors to prescribe rest, meditation and a one- or two-week spa vacation to rest and rejuvenate the body. We need to return to this way of thinking. Any injury or disease requires time for the tissues to heal.

When you injure your back or neck and find functioning difficult, take one day off from work. Rest, apply cold therapy and use some anti-inflammatory medication if prescribed by your doctor. While you are resting, do not anguish over the time you are missing from work. Instead think about what elements of your lifestyle are out of balance and could have contributed to your injury. Rest, relaxation and reflection are usually better than medication.

MEDICATION

There are many over-the-counter anti-inflammatories and analgesics (painkillers) to help you in times of need. Research clearly demonstrates that anti-inflammatory medication is superior to painkillers at getting you back to work after a neck or back injury. Medications such as Advil, Nuprin, Motrin, Aleve and aspirin are usually safe and effective. Always read the literature which lists directions and warnings and talk to your doctor if you use these products more than occasionally or in conjunction with other medication.

Some people are not able to take one or more of these medications. If you have any questions at all about the use of a medication, you should consult your medical doctor for advice on an anti-inflammatory that is right for you.

THE THERAPEUTIC CANE

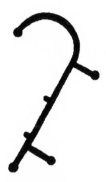

The therapeutic cane, or Thera-Cane, is a device that I have used successfully with thousands of patients. This device is used once or twice per day, by placing gentle sustained pressure on tight, sensitive muscles. Using this device for approximately :60 seconds in the morning or evening can dramatically lessen muscular aches and pains. If you find yourself feeling increased soreness from this device, you are either doing it too hard or too frequently. This device is most effective on the upper back, middle back, lower back and legs. Follow the exercises in the appendix at the end of the book to learn how to properly use the Thera-Cane to massage the head, neck and front of your body.

Figure 19-1.
The Thera-Cane

:60 SECOND SELF MASSAGE: THE SENSITIVE SPOTS

Use the following :60 second techniques when you want to release stress in any of your five stress zones.

Zones 1 and Zone 2: Facing the World

Use the fingertips of both hands to gently massage your scalp, forehead and facial muscles. Make gentle circles in both directions and continue until you feel a relief from the pressure and tension. Be certain that you massage the nose, the area around the eyes and any area which you habitually contract in your first stress zone.

The muscles that open and close your jaw are some of the

strongest muscles in the body. Stress and tension can cause chronic pressure and pain in this area, which can radiate into your face, throughout your jaw, into your ears and down your neck. To help relieve some of this pressure, start massaging at the top of these muscles, just below the ridge of bone which runs from the middle of your ear towards the edge of your eye. Below this ridge you will feel thick ropy muscles which extend down, vertically, to the angle of your jaw. Massage these muscles with your fingertips in a circular motion or rub across them as if you were strumming the strings of a guitar. Do both sides and continue until you feel your jaw bone relax. Then massage the area around your mouth and along your throat and neck.

Zone 3: Opening the Chest

This is the area which corresponds to your third stress zone and consists of the upper back and chest. The following techniques are extremely successful at relieving stress and tension in these areas. Make a gentle fist and reach behind and across your upper body, to your opposite shoulder. For example, your left fist would contact your right upper back. Strike the upper back muscles with the base of your thumb as the primary contact point. Do this three to five times and then strike the other shoulder. This type of pounding massage technique is called *tapotement* and is quite effective at softening spasm and increasing circulation. You may also use the palm half of your fist to gently strike the muscles in your chest and upper arms. You may also massage your chest muscles by using your fingertips to rub these chest muscles in a circular motion concentrating on the two pads of muscles on either side of your sternum.

Zone 4: Organizing Your Organs

Your stomach, intestines, liver, spleen, gall bladder and kidneys are all located in your abdominal cavity. Researchers at a major British hospital and medical center, after having studied chronic stomach pain, concluded that most common stomach and abdominal symptoms were from muscular tension. This technique is an extremely effective method of relieving muscular tension and can eliminate many types of mild to moderate abdominal complaints.

Lie on your back with your knees up and your feet flat on the floor. Putting a small amount of cream or oil on your stomach, gently use your fingers and palm to massage your stomach in a clockwise motion. Because your food moves through the intestines in a clockwise direction, avoid massaging counter-clockwise. Massage for approximately :60 seconds, working in small and large circles, as if you were tracing the concentric rings of a bull's-eye. Continue until you feel a relief of pressure and tension.

Zone 5: The Forbidden City

Use your fingertips to gently massage your lower abdominal region, pubis and genitals. The muscles on the inside of your thighs should also be included. Because the muscles in this region are quite sensitive, they will require a lighter touch and less time than the thick, commonly contracted muscles in your upper back, neck and shoulders.

WHEN TO CALL A DOCTOR

If you have pain which is not improving after twenty-four to forty-eight hours, call your physician right away. Also, immediately call your doctor if the pain begins to radiate down your arm or leg or if the pain is extremely acute. Any pain which persists or becomes moderate to severe may indicate a serious problem.

:60 SECOND PAIN MANAGEMENT SUMMARY

- Cold should be used to treat any new or acute injury (and when there is inflammation) before ever considering heat.
- Heat should be used to treat older, chronic and milder problems.
- Rest really is the best medicine—force yourself to rest after sustaining an injury.
- Take anti-inflammatories when appropriate (check with your doctor).
- Call your physician if pain doesn't decrease after twenty-four to forty-eight hours.
- Tissue heals, but muscle remembers.
- Try using the Thera-Cane, following the exercises in the appendix.
- Massage each of the five stress zones as described in this chapter.

Chapter 20

CANCER AND DIET—
THEORIES AND ANSWERS

:60 Second Affirmation:
"I eat food that aids and protects my health."

I will never forget John's face when he walked into my office in 1995. His face was slightly ashen and his mood downcast. He told me that he was sixty-nine years old and had little to look forward to. Six months earlier he suffered the ravages of a triple bypass heart operation. Just as he was beginning to recover from this traumatic surgery, he was given bad news. The middle back pain which I had not been able to fix was diagnosed as cancer.

John looked me in the eyes and said quite sincerely, "If I had known I was going to live this long, I would have taken better care of myself." All I could do for John at that moment was to help him gently bring closure to his life. After fifty years of smoking cigarettes, eating charbroiled steaks and avoiding fruits and vegetables, he had irreparably damaged his body. John's typical breakfast consisted of bacon or sausage, eggs and two or three cups of coffee. Lunch usually consisted of a hamburger and French fries, washed down by a couple of soft drinks. His late afternoon pick-me-up snack was a candy bar and a couple more cups of coffee, just enough caffeine and chocolate to get him through the day.

When he arrived home after a long day at the office, John would drink a few glasses of whiskey, have a steak for dinner with a couple of glasses of wine, always avoiding, as he put it, anything green. Or he would eat a baked potato *drenched with butter and sour cream as his only vegetable for the entire day. Then he was too tired to exercise so he would sit in front of the television, and often knock off a quart of full fat ice cream while watching his favorite sitcom. Before retiring for bed, he would smoke his last cigarette, after having consumed one to two packs that day.*

John passed away six months after our last visit as the cancer metastasized rapidly through his system. Unlike John, most of us get a second chance. I wished I had had a chance to talk to John twenty years earlier. But it is not too late for most of the rest of us, despite age or physical condition, to improve our health, outlook and lifestyle.

Say the word cancer and many people shudder. The fear of cancer is deeply ingrained in us. Everyone has a friend, a loved one, a relative or a neighbor who has succumbed to this deadly disease. In fact, news of a rapid and sudden death from a massive heart attack seems less threatening. While a heart attack is a swift killer, cancer often leads to a slow, lingering and painful death. Watching a loved one slowly waste away from cancer is enough to make anyone fearful of this deadly disease. But there is something you can do about it.

Recent research theorizes that one cancer-causing component is poor diet. There is no question that for some people, a high risk for cancer seems to run in their families. Whether this is due to heredity or environment is uncertain. You have little control over your heredity; however, you do have some control over your environment—and, more importantly, a tremendous amount of control over what you eat.

We are constantly bombarded by hundreds of diets supposedly recommended to reduce the risk of cancer. Carrots have been touted, low-fat diets promoted, fish oil heralded. The wide variety of experts espousing their various philosophies makes it difficult to discern opinion from truth based upon solid scientific research.

RECENT CANCER DIET RESEARCH

Researchers from the University of California at Berkeley did extensive research into the causes of cancer. They concluded that, as cancer preventatives, we should do the following:
1. Stop smoking.
2. Control infections.
3. Avoid intense sun exposure.
4. Reduce alcohol consumption.
5. Reduce red meat intake.

These researchers concluded that pollution, pesticides and stress had the lowest impact upon the likelihood of developing cancer. They clearly noted that cigarettes are a potent carcinogen and repeated infections can create local cell damage which may, in some cases, turn into cancer.

They did not recommend that people completely stop consuming alcohol or red meat. Their research concluded that drinking alcohol and eating meat in moderation were not associated with an increase in the likelihood of developing cancer. Most importantly, these Berkeley experts touted two factors as being most important in preventing cancer:

1. Eating plenty of fresh fruits and vegetables.
2. Getting plenty of exercise.

Our primitive forefathers ate mostly fruits and vegetables and were physically active. The :60 Second Rejuvenation Strategy is completely in agreement with this modern scientific research. For example, foods included in the :60 Second Rejuvenation diet, like spinach, garlic, tomatoes, red grapes, whole grains, and fish, were among those on a recently published list of the top ten foods to help fight cancer.

STEAK VERSUS BROCCOLI

Some health food advocates exhort the necessity of completely avoiding meat, fish and chicken. They defend the philosophy that only a strict vegetarian diet will promote health and longevity and prevent cancer. But recent research contradicts this theory.

The Fred Hutchinson Cancer Research Center published a study in 1999 which concluded that some types of individuals may have a slightly elevated risk for certain types of cancer if they eat excessive amounts of processed or overly-cooked meats. Highly salted meats, packaged and processed lunch meats and charred steaks may not be ideal foods, but they concluded that these meats, eaten in small quantities, were quite safe. If you decide to eat beef, pork or any other meat for that matter, try baking or broiling it rather than frying. Baking or broiling meat allows the fat to drip off and avoids the blackened appearance which may be less healthy.

Scientists in Sweden recently came to a startling discovery. Their research, published in the journal Appetite in April, 1999, concluded that meat consumption was not necessarily a cause of cancer and coronary heart disease. This interesting investigation noted that people who ate a lot of meat tended to eat less poultry, fish, fruit, cereals and cheese. Their study of almost 12,000 people noted no major association between meat eating and cholesterol level, nor was there any relationship to the likelihood of getting cancer. Although eating meat may not be the problem, a deficiency in other necessary nutrients may be.

Recommendations on dietary practices that prevent cancer have been published recently by the prestigious American Institute for Cancer Research and the World Cancer Research Fund. They concluded that people's diets should be based on plant products, primarily emphasizing fruits and vegetables, supplemented with beans, legumes and small portions of fish and poultry. They concluded that by limiting the intake of sugary foods, cured or smoked meats and deep fried foods, people could decrease their chances of developing cancer.

Similarly, scientists at Rutgers University concluded that even our three-million-year-old ancestor, *Australopithecus*, subsisted on fruits, vegetables, leaves and high quality animal foods. Even before the Stone Age, our ancestors were eating lean meats, fruits and vegetables.

If you think you have any form of cancer, you must consult a medical physician immediately. Curing cancer is a difficult proposition. Preventing cancer is far easier to accomplish. Anti-cancer diets include plenty of fresh fruits and vegetables and whole grains. Onions and garlic and regular exercise have also been proven to be anti-cancer agents. Avoid junk foods and processed meats, as well as harmful pesticides and chemicals. Always wash your fruits and vegetables well before eating. Try to avoid unnecessary or excessive x-rays and drink plenty of green tea. Regular exercise, a low-fat diet and plenty of fruits and vegetables are important. They may prevent or help you deal with cancer.

:60 SECOND CANCER/DIET ADVICE SUMMARY

- Recent research suggests that one cancer causing component may be poor diet.
- Eating meat does not appear to be related to getting cancer.
- Eat fresh fruits and vegetables, supplemented with beans and legumes, to prevent cancer says the American Institute for Cancer Research and World Cancer Research Fund.
- Stop smoking, control infections, avoid intense sun exposure and reduce alcohol consumption as cancer preventatives.
- Do not eat large quantities of highly salted or smoked meats, packaged or processed lunch meats or blackened steak.
- Limit intake of sugary foods and deep-fried foods.
- Follow our ancestors—eat lean meats, fruits and vegetables.
- Get plenty of exercise.

Chapter 21

AGING—REJUVENATION, NOT DEGENERATION

:60 Second Affirmation:
"We turn not older with years, but newer every day."
Emily Dickinson

When Laura entered my office, all eyes shifted towards her. Bubbly and talkative, she commanded the attention of all around her. No one could believe she was eighty-two years old. Her short stature and curly gray hair masked the heart of a teenager. I attributed Laura's good health to her commitment to regular exercise, daily meditation and a healthy diet.

Laura grew up in France during World War II and rarely had enough to eat. After the war Laura came to the United States to study English and decided to stay. Although she missed her family, she felt exhilarated being away from the political chaos and rubble caused by the war with Germany. Laura's first job was as a ticket seller in the circus. Enchanted by the excitement and color of circus life, Laura studied with many of the performers. Her terrific sense of timing and drama impressed her tutors, and she was hired as a fire eater and lion tamer. Laura spoke fondly of her fifteen years as a circus performer and how she fell in love with and married a trapeze artist, eventually giving birth to three sons. But Laura's first husband died in a trapeze accident and her second husband died in a fiery car crash. Laura needed a more stable life for her three children. She left the circus and worked as a secretary, a job she pursued for the next twenty years. Although it lacked the glamour of the circus, it provided the

140

security needed to support a family. While living in Los Angeles she began searching for more spiritual meaning. Having abandoned Catholicism, she soon discovered an affinity for yoga and meditation.

Although Laura was quite healthy, she suffered from mild, chronic neck and hip pain which she attributed to years of circus injuries. Her yoga and med-itation were not able to relieve her of these nagging aches. During her first ses-sion with me, she comically described to me how she and all of her retired friends suffered from arthritis. "Doc," she said, "when you're over seventy and you wake up in the morning without pain, you know you're dead!" Then she added, "But it's better to wear out than to rust out." After performing only a few sessions of gentle stretching and massage on her neck and hip and providing her with some very specific exercises, she said she felt nearly pain-free.

Laura would often come to my office with very minor complaints and explained that when the big pains go away, you always feel the little ones. I will never forget that phrase. In fact, it has become an important part of the :60 Second Rejuvenation Strategy. Laura taught me that the path to high-level well-ness demanded working on the biggest health problems first. Then, with time, you can focus on more subtle issues. Becoming healthy requires getting rid of the larger problems first and then focusing on the little ones.

Dean Ornish, a medical doctor at the University of California, San Francisco Medical Center has proven that a healthy lifestyle can not only prevent deterioration, it can actually reverse it. Dr. Ornish asked patients with heart disease to walk briskly three times per week, practice relaxation and breathing techniques, meditation and eat a low-fat high-fiber diet. When he performed MRI scans of the arteries of these individuals he found that this program could actually reverse the thick, fatty plaques in the coronary arteries. Also they had lower cho-lesterol, lower blood pressure and a better outlook on life.

At almost any age you can reverse the negative effects caused by trauma, years of unhealthy habits and the ravages of illness. But you must be willing to change your lifestyle and follow new guidelines. Although we do not know exactly how nutrition affects longevity, we do know a tremendous amount about the relationship between nutrition and aging.

Researchers at Tufts University in Boston recently concluded that a diet emphasizing vegetables was correlated with low body fat in the elderly. They noted that desserts, snack foods and a high carbohy-drate intake was associated with increased weight gain and poor health. This is important because a person who is overweight has an increased chance of injury during exercise, as well as a higher incidence of many kinds of health problems.

A healthy diet not only reduces the risk of developing disease and obesity, it also helps prevent cancer and a variety of other diseases and delays aging. Aging and cancer appear to be directly related, in good part, to production of toxins produced by our own cells. These toxins or *oxidants* are produced by *mitochondria*, small structures inside of every cell. Mitochondria generate oxidants as a byproduct of their normal metabolism. Preventing the spread of oxidants throughout your body will prevent rapid aging and many types of illness.

You have probably seen advertisements for *anti-oxidant supplements*, touting them as being necessary for good health. Although there is some evidence that supplementing your diet with these vitamins, minerals and nutrients will improve health, there is even more evidence proving that natural foods, especially fruits and vegetables, produce the most profound anti-aging and anti-cancer effects.

The University of California at Berkeley, an important research center in the field of health and human aging, published a report concluding that many kinds of nutrients could actually prevent cancer and delay aging. They concluded that the nutrients in fresh fruits and vegetables had a significant protective effect. They also noted that vitamins B_{12}, B_6 and folic deficiencies were also more common in patients with cancer and concluded that these nutritional deficits could actually damage DNA, the basic building blocks of your genes.

Because your chromosomes act to guide and direct all body processes, any problems in their performance can have profound negative consequences. These researchers also observed that deficiencies in these nutrients caused damage by a mechanism quite similar to the damage caused by radiation and chemicals. Even the European Cancer Prevention Organization, which studied mortality data over a twenty-year period, concluded that fruits and vegetables had protective effects against cancer and other types of degenerative diseases.

The University of Minnesota School of Public Health published an article in 1999 which compared older women who ate whole grain products with those who ate refined grain products. The elderly women eating the natural foods had far better health and longevity than those who ate refined gains, such as white bread and pasta. Aging gracefully does not require that you go on a spartan diet consisting of only produce.

An article in the *Journal of the American Medical Association* reported on a study done at Harvard School of Public Health that examined the eating habits of more than 100,000 seniors and middle-aged individuals looking for a relationship between egg consumption and disease. They concluded that even eating one egg per day would be unlikely to have any harmful effects. This well-documented research report could find no significant relationship between eating eggs and cholesterol or heart disease. As you age, you will need sufficient protein, vitamins, minerals and fats to remain healthy. Eggs are a great addition to a diet primarily composed of fruits, vegetables and whole grains. Just don't smother those scrambled eggs in butter and cheddar cheese.

Another Australian study made an international comparison of food intake among the aged. Their study of approximately 2,000 elderly people concluded that a diet rich in plant foods, in particular vegetables, legumes and fruit, protected these seniors against premature death. Results from the study also noted that a high intake of seafood and lean meats and a low intake of fatty meats was also important. Thus, modern international research on the relationship of diet to health is in complete agreement with the principles outlined in the :60 Second Rejuvenation Strategy. Seniors should emphasize eating fresh fruits and vegetables, supplemented by lean fish and chicken. Eggs, nuts, seeds and whole grains should be added because they are valuable sources of protein, vitamins, minerals and trace elements. The diet of our ancestors, with its emphasis upon natural foods, is appropriate for modern day people of all ages, especially seniors.

Many older people live alone and find it difficult to shop—or even forget to eat. Before shopping, seniors need to remember the :60 Second Rejuvenation Strategy shopping tip: Always go to the fruit and vegetable section first, then buy lean meats, followed by whole grains and then everything else. Whether you are a senior or not, writing down a list of items needed can save time and ensure that you will follow the :60 Second Rejuvenation Strategy. By following the strategy, you will naturally consume the proper balance of vitamins, minerals, protein, fats and sodium.

BONING UP ON SUPPLEMENTS

Osteoporosis, or thinning bones, is a common problem in old age. This can cause spinal curvature, hip or vertebral fracture or loss of teeth. To preserve your bones you need to have a sufficient supply of calcium, Vitamin D and other minerals. Be certain that you take a multivitamin, multimineral supplement daily and follow the :60 Second Rejuvenation Strategy diet. Make sure that you eat plenty of fish and lean chicken and supplement your diet with low-fat dairy products. Canned salmon and sardines, tofu and low-fat cottage cheese are other foods which provide large amounts of calcium and are low in fat.

Try to avoid drinking more than two cups of coffee or alcohol per day, as it can increase the risk of osteoporosis. Cigarettes and many prescription drugs can also contribute to osteoporosis. Rather than drinking large amounts of coffee, alcohol or soda, try drinking more water. Research published in the journal, *Gerontology*, in 1999 suggested that the elderly may recognize thirst less readily than younger individuals. By drinking plenty of fresh water, juice and green tea you will slow down aging, increase vitality and reduce the risk of cancer and other serious illnesses.

MATURE, BUT FIT

Our ancient ancestors did not have to worry about sweating on a stair climber or grunting while performing push-ups. Exercise, especially walking and lifting, was part of their everyday routine. By comparison, we have become lazy. Most of us spend our day sitting at a desk or in front of a computer and then sit in the evening to read the newspaper or watch television. You can quickly rejuvenate even years of laziness.

A study published in 1998 by the Advanced Research Center for Human Sciences in Japan produced some very interesting results. They found that in less than three months, after lifting weights three times per week, the average improvement in strength in older adults was thirty-five to forty percent. They also found that the seniors reported improved mood, decreased anxiety and an overall sense of psychological well-being. The average age of this group was about sixty-nine years old.

Seniors need to start exercising gently, approximately five to ten minutes, twice a week. Slowly add increased time and vigor as you become more comfortable with your routine. The simplest, safest exercises to strengthen the heart, lungs and bones are walking and lifting light weights. There is no need to join a gym. One- to two-pound dumbbells and light ankle weights provide enough resistance to increase your level of fitness. Swimming, yoga and gentle stretching exercises are also safe and easy to perform. Luckily, you don't need to kill yourself to receive benefits from exercise.

Another study published in the *Journal of Cardiovascular Risk* studied the cholesterol of middle-aged men and concluded that moderate exercise was as effective as the highly stressful routines of the elite athlete. The stretching exercises suggested in the *:60 Second Rejuvenation*

Strategy are quite simple and easy to perform. They provide an excellent routine for the active older adult. Add the Kegel exercises to help improve bladder control. Other aerobic activities can also be beneficial. Bicycling, dancing and running in place are all safe and effective ways of increasing your level of fitness. Hiking, stair stepping and walking on an indoor treadmill are other good alternatives.

SEXY SENIORS

Although some sexual function declines with age, sexual ability is more of a function of physical fitness than anything else. A study done at Stanford University School of Medicine concluded that there was a high level of sexual activity and satisfaction in some men and women over fifty. One very interesting conclusion was the correlation between sexual satisfaction and the degree of physical fitness. They concluded that physical fitness and high levels of sexual activity are mutually supportive elements in aging.

Growing old does not mean that you do not have sex, but one must be prepared for a slightly different style. A study performed by the University of Massachusetts Medical Center also concluded that smoking and excessive alcohol consumption reduced the hormones responsible for sex drive. Generally, older men require more gentle manual stimulation of the penis and a longer period prior to getting an erection. A regular pattern of sexual activity helps to preserve this ability. Increased body awareness and masturbation all help to preserve sexual ability. Although drugs such as Viagra can help improve sexual function, it is important to realize that many physical problems, such as hypertension, heart disease and diabetes can make sexuality more difficult. Other drugs such as steroids, blood pressure medication and analgesics can also reduce sex drive. Women may find that their vagina may feel tight or dry. This can be overcome with a vaginal lubricant, Kegel exercises and a slow resumption of sexual activity.

WRINKLES, WEALTH AND WISDOM

Each chapter of life can bring its own satisfaction. Retirement can bring with it less stress and more enjoyable leisure time activities. Becoming involved in church and charity functions can provide mental stimulation and gratification. Yes, there is a downside. Chronic pain, loneliness and approaching death can be depressing. However, staying involved and active are effective ways of making the golden years productive and happy.

Luckily, now research is conclusive that a good diet with regular physical exercise and plenty of relaxation is the perfect antidote to depression. Many natural therapies which include herbs, massage and homeopathy have been shown to be helpful in cases of mild to moderate depression. However, if natural therapies are not enough, you might need to see a psychologist or psychiatrist. Sleep problems, loss of appetite, overwhelming sadness or pain and forgetfulness can be helped by medication as well as behavior modification.

STRAIGHTENING OUT YOUR LIFE

Proper body alignment is an integral part of the :60 Second Rejuvenation Strategy. Without proper posture, you will slump, disturbing your body's natural balance, making it easier to fall and cause injury. If your friends have commented on your increasing slump or you have been shocked by your appearance in the mirror, it is time to start practicing your postural exercises. The exercises in the :60 Second Rejuvenation Strategy are gentle, simple and easy to perform. Spend a few minutes each day trying to find your ideal neutral or natural position.

MATURITY AND SPIRITUAL GROWTH

A study performed at Duke University Medical Center's Department of Psychiatry concluded that seniors with high levels of trust were healthier and more optimistic about life. These findings illustrate the rejuvenating effects of a positive outlook. In India, it is accepted that the first half of your life is spent with your work and family and the second half is devoted to spiritual growth. Meditation and prayer are important foundations to spiritual and religious growth. Regular visits to your church or temple can provide not only an uplifting spiritual experience, but also a network of friends and acquaintances. As you age, your temple or church congregation can provide a second family if your own children have grown up or moved away. Early civilizations built their towns around the church or temple. Our primitive ancestors knew that a deep relationship with higher spiritual powers promoted health, wellness and a sense of community.

Your style of meditation or prayer may need to be modified as you age. Kneeling in a church pew or sitting cross-legged on the floor can be difficult as your joints stiffen. Prayer and meditation is easily performed sitting in a comfortable chair or even in bed. Remember that work, love and spiritual growth are the foundation of a healthy life.

:60 SECOND MATURITY REJUVENATION SUMMARY

• Maintaining a healthy diet as you age not only reduces the risk of developing disease and obesity, it also helps prevent cancer and delays the effects of aging.

• Your aging body will need sufficient protein, vitamins, minerals and fats to remain healthy.

• Drinking plenty of fresh water, juice and green tea will slow down aging, increase vitality and reduce the risk of cancer and other serious illnesses.

• The simplest, safest exercises to strengthen the heart, lungs and bones of mature people are walking and lifting light weights.

• Proper body alignment is an integral part of the *:60 Second Rejuvenation Strategy.*

• Regular visits to your church or temple can provide not only an uplifting spiritual experience in your senior years, but also a network of friends and acquaintances.

• Remember that work, love and spiritual growth—the three parts of the healthy triangle—are the foundation of a healthy life no matter what your age.

Chapter 22

COMMON AILMENTS—
PROVEN TREATMENTS

:60 Second Affirmation:
"With education I can avoid medication."

Victor, *a sixty-two-year-old retired psychologist, was an avid reader. He had always entered my office with a magazine or book nestled under his arm. Victor researched every ailment he had and would question his doctors about each therapy they suggested. For colds, he took echinacea, garlic and golden seal. Bouts of back pain sent him running off to yoga teachers, massage therapists and chiropractors. I attributed his good health to his desire to understand common ailments and all of the medical as well as complimentary therapies available.*

Victor was the Western States Tennis Champion in the "Sixty years and older" age group. There was no doubt in my mind that his physical and mental vigor were due to his incredible perseverance to understand disease, medical therapies and high-level wellness. I was saddened when Victor came to my office complaining of chronic leg pain.

Two months of spinal mobilization, anti-inflammatory medication and exercise brought no relief. I referred Victor to an orthopedic medical doctor who sent him out for an MRI and concluded that he suffered from a severe case of spinal stenosis, an excessive degeneration of the spinal column, causing bone to grow around vital nerves, creating serious and incapacitating leg pain. The doctor recommended injections of cortisone to help him cope with the pain and physical therapy to help him learn to stretch out the chronic muscle spasm in his leg. Neither treatment relieved his debilitating condition. I referred him to an acupuncturist, which he found somewhat helpful, but Victor was still suffering. I decided to refer him to a spinal surgeon.

A few weeks later, he returned to my office. He told me that he had seen five spinal surgeons–all recommended surgery immediately. I wished Victor good luck and prayed for a positive result. I wondered about Victor but I hesitated to call him, worried that, at his age, the outcome of such a radical surgery was unpredictable. Six months later, Victor came bounding into my office with his athletic stride and in his freshly starched tennis outfit. I asked him how the surgery had gone. To my amazement he told me that he never had the surgery! He continued to have acupuncture and perform his home exercises and eventually the pain was alleviated. Victor told me that he had done further research on his problem and discovered that, in a small number of cases, spinal stenosis would spontaneously disappear. He reasoned that eventually his compressed nerves could adapt to bony impingement if the inflammation was reduced and the nerves were stretched to make them more flexible. Acupuncture, anti-inflammatory medication and exercise had created a medical miracle. But the magic was not in the combination of therapies–it was the faith Victor had in his ability to understand and cure his own illness. Being fully informed about alternative therapies and medical procedures had helped Victor avoid the possible serious side effects of spinal surgery.

Many common ailments respond to natural therapies. These therapies can help to relieve illness while improving your health. They can rejuvenate mind, body and spirit. Always check with your doctor so that you are certain that your symptoms are not due to a more serious illness. There are times when you must seek out the help of a trained professional.

ALLERGIES

Signs of food allergy such as a runny nose, wheezing, gas, swollen joints, coughing and a general feeling of malaise are very common. It is possible to be allergic to almost any food, such as bread, pastry, dairy products, some nuts and shellfish which are common provocateurs of these symptoms. If your allergic reaction is minor, you can easily determine which food is causing it by trying to eliminate the food you suspect for three days, eating only vegetables, rice and chicken. Then, eat the potentially allergic food and notice its effect. Many people report that after one or two servings, they are clearly aware of their allergies.

Another strategy involves taking your pulse a few minutes after eating a potentially allergic food. If your pulse rate increases by more than ten additional beats per minute, this may also be indicative of an allergic reaction. Some people find that stress reduction, taking multivitamins and herbs are quite helpful. Try a combination of stinging nettle and goldenseal. They can help offset the effects of seasonal allergies. If your allergies persist, see your doctor. If you are allergic to a particular food, a modification of your diet is essential.

ARTERIOSCLEROSIS

Arteriosclerosis involves the building up of thick, fatty deposits on your arteries and veins. This condition can increase the likelihood of heart disease and stroke. There is no question that eating a diet primarily consisting of fruits and vegetables is an excellent antidote. To prevent arteriosclerosis, pile your plate high with fresh fruits and vegetables and supplement this with lean meats and poultry. Regular vigorous exercise also helps keep your arteries clear. There is some proof that garlic and hawthorne are excellent herbs for preventing and managing heart disease. Always see your doctor if you suspect any type of heart problem.

BACK AND NECK PAIN

Solving back and neck pain can be accomplished by following the prescription outlined in the :60 Second Rejuvenation Strategy. Use proper body alignment and get regular gentle exercise, including stretching, strengthening and aerobics. Glucosamine sulfate and chondroitin sulfate have been shown to improve the health of your cartilage. Gentle chiropractic manipulation can also improve range of motion, and acupuncture can reduce inflammation. If the pain persists, see a doctor.

COLDS AND FLU

If you are suffering from sneezing, mild fever, runny nose, head congestion, with many types of minor aches and pains, you are probably suffering from the common cold. A cold is a mild upper respiratory viral infection. Many people report that echinacea, goldenseal and garlic are quite helpful. Vitamin C has also been shown to be beneficial. You might find that avoiding all dairy products and wheat significantly limits mucus production and head congestion. If your mucus is green or red or the cold persists for more than a few days, check with your doctor to rule out a more serious infection.

DEPRESSION

If you feel tired, lack motivation and the world seems bleak, you may be suffering from depression. Many people feel more depressed throughout the winter, during times of increased stress or after any dramatic life-changing event. St. John's wort, a balanced diet, plenty of sunlight, multivitamin or mineral supplements and regular exercise can all relieve the effects of depression. If the systems persist or you feel suicidal, be sure to see your doctor or contact a mental health professional.

HEART DISEASE

If you suffer from chest pain, shortness of breath or pain down your arm, be sure to see your doctor immediately. You should regularly visit a physician if you are overweight, or have a family history of heart problems or high cholesterol. Hawthorne is an herb which has been proven to stabilize uneven heart rate. A diet rich in fruits and vegetables, regular aerobic exercise and meditation can all reduce the risk of developing heart problems. Research also indicates that eating fish, supplementing your diet with plenty of garlic and drinking green tea can help reduce the likelihood of getting heart disease.

INSOMNIA AND SLEEP DISORDERS

If you wake up many times during the night, have difficulty falling asleep or wake up too early, you may be suffering from some form of insomnia. Valerian, passionflower and kava kava are herbs that can help induce a good night's sleep. Stress reduction techniques, having a regular bedtime and proper diet are all helpful. If your sleep problem becomes serious, be sure to check with your doctor. Some sleep problems can be due to an underlying metabolic disorder.

MENOPAUSE

If you are a woman over forty years old suffering from hot flashes, heart palpitations, depression and dizziness, you may be suffering from menopause. This can last up to five years and can be quite distressing. Many women report that evening primrose oil, black cohosh, vitex (or chaste berry) and dong quay can be helpful. Regular exercise, meditation and a good night's sleep are important. If the symptoms persist, see your doctor and ask about hormone therapy which may include taking estrogen and/or progesterone.

OBESITY

If you are twenty percent or more over the average weight for your height and build, you may have excess fat. Obesity puts a tremendous amount of stress on your heart and lungs, as well as all of your joints. Regular exercise and a low-fat diet are the ideal solutions. A hormonal disorder can also cause you to gain a tremendous amount of weight. Check with your doctor if diet and exercise do not solve your problem.

OSTEOPOROSIS

Osteoporosis is the gradual loss of minerals from your bones. There is no question that regular weight-bearing exercise such as walking and gentle weight lifting can be effective. Supplement your diet daily with 1,000 to 2,000 milligrams of calcium daily in the form of a multivitamin/mineral supplement. Every woman fifty years and older should be checked by a physician for osteoporosis.

SINUSITIS

Frequent headaches, pressure behind the eyes and regular postnasal drip can be signs of sinusitis. This refers to an inflammation in the sinuses which are located above and below your eyes. Because this can become an infection, try to treat it as soon as possible. Avoiding wheat and dairy products and using a salt water nasal spray three times per day can be helpful.

STOMACH AND INTESTINAL PROBLEMS

Diarrhea, constipation, gas and indigestion can be an annoyance. Drinking mint or ginger tea can help soothe a queasy stomach. Licorice root supplements can be helpful, especially if they are the type with the glycyrrhizic acid removed. Acupuncture and stress reduction techniques will also help calm an upset stomach. If your symptoms persist, see your doctor right away. Chronic stomach problems or a significant change in bowel habits can indicate a more serious disorder.

STRESS AND ANXIETY

Stress is a part of everyday life. However, if your stress level rises to a point where you have difficulty functioning in work and/or social situations, you may have a problem. Look at your job, your marriage or love relationships, your financial situation and other major life changes. Increased difficulty at work and family problems are the most common causes. Proper diet, regular exercise and meditation are extremely important. Herbs such as valerian, kava kava and passionflower reduce anxiety. Try drinking less caffeinated beverages and substituting some chamomile tea. Decaffeinated coffees and teas can also be an alternative if you have trouble giving up these potent and satisfying brews. Above all, get plenty of rest and exercise, eat well, and see a therapist or physician if your symptoms persist.

:60 SECOND COMMON AILMENT MANAGEMENT SUMMARY

- Many common ailments respond to natural therapy.
- Always consult a physician before beginning new regimens.
- If you are allergic to a particular food, modification of your diet is essential.
- Eating a diet primarily consisting of fresh fruits and vegetables is an excellent antidote and preventative for many diseases.
- Curing many illnesses can be difficult; preventing them is often far easier.
- Mental illnesses as well as physical illnesses respond to a balanced diet and regular exercise.
- Every woman fifty years and older should be checked by a physician for osteoporosis.

Chapter 23

COMPLIMENTARY MEDICINE—
ALTERNATIVE CARE

:60 Second Affirmation:
"From nature, to nature"

I was surprised when Ralph, a noted physician in my community, as well as a professor at the nearby prestigious medical center, came into my office. Ralph had developed chronic neck pain that had not been cured by medication or physical therapy. His colleagues had prescribed numerous anti-inflammatory regimens to cure his problem. These drugs created a bleeding stomach ulcer, a side-effect of the medication. Fifteen physical therapy sessions later, he was still suffering from chronic neck pain. Ralph asked his physician friends for the name of a good chiropractor. Although many of his colleagues scoffed at his question, two of them, who were my patients, gave him my card. Ralph called my office that day for an appointment.

After examining Ralph, I concluded that his neck pain was caused by osteoarthritis, a chronic degenerative disc and joint disorder. I told Ralph that this disease had caused the vertebrae in his neck to stiffen, creating chronic pain. I asked him to come to my office for three treatments of gentle joint stretching and prescribed a home exercise program. He quickly agreed.

Ralph showed up for his appointments, performed his exercises religiously and did not question my suggestions. Luckily for both of us, three sessions of therapy cured the majority of his neck problem. Ralph was very surprised that the *results were so dramatic. Before discharging him, I asked him how he felt about complimentary medicine. Ralph responded, "Being a scientist necessitates investigating every possible avenue." He continued, "Especially after my experience with you, I feel that doctors who do not investigate alternative medicine with an open mind are unscientific and biased." Ralph went on to tell me that he felt that both medical doctors who criticize alternative medicine and healers who shun drugs and surgery are quacks. Ralph understood that some maladies respond best to complimentary therapies and more serious problems require medical intervention.*

Although the *:60 Second Rejuvenation Strategy* can be seen as a guide to health and well-being, there are times when expert advice is needed. Because your medical doctor has the broadest access to diagnostic tools, he/she should be the first person you turn to for help. Medical doctors have a close working relationship with hospitals and have the best training in diagnosing a wide variety of illness. However, most doctors use a very limited number of therapies. They usually limit their practice to drugs and surgery.

In some cases, drugs and surgery are the treatment of choice and are effective. For example, it is not wise to treat a serious infection with natural therapy. An infection can spread throughout the body, causing serious injury or death. Luckily, many health problems are not serious and respond well to natural therapy. Natural therapies are also referred to as *complimentary medicine* or *alternative medicine*. I prefer the term *complimentary medicine*, because I feel that natural and medical therapies compliment each other, each having their own strengths and weaknesses. The more educated you are on natural therapies, the more choice you'll have if you need treatment for an illness or condition. It is vital that you are aware of all of the options available to you before you begin any course of treatment.

The following natural therapies are rooted in primitive healing traditions and can be considered as an adjunct to your personal health care.

ACUPUNCTURE—NEEDLES AND ROOTS

Acupuncture has been around for almost 5,000 years. It is widely accepted throughout China, Korea and Japan, and is growing in popularity throughout the United States, Europe and much of Latin America. The primary therapy provided by acupuncturists involves the insertion of tiny needles into specific points in the skin and/or prescribing herbs. The acupuncturist believes that the acupuncture needles and the herbal medicine can modify your life force to remedy many illnesses. Acupuncturists also use nutritional counseling and massage in their practice. Acupuncture appears to be most effective when used to treat back and neck pain, muscle spasms and headaches. Many people also find it helpful for digestive problems, stress and a wide range of mild illnesses.

Although acupuncture is a very effective therapy, it should not be utilized with a serious illness unless you have first seen your medical doctor. Acupuncture is generally safe and can be of great benefit in certain cases, but make sure that your acupuncturist utilizes disposable needles and is up to date on the side effects of herbal medicine. If the thought of acupuncture conjures up visions of pincushions or potentially dangerous herbal remedies, try *acupressure massage* first. A massage therapist can provide gentle pressure to acupuncture points, creating similar results.

CHIROPRACTIC—IS IT ALL IT'S CRACKED UP TO BE?

Most chiropractors loosen your spinal joints by providing manipulation or adjustments. Although there are many chiropractic schools of thought, most chiropractors provide some type of manipulation, massage and exercise therapy.

One of the most widely respected studies of chiropractic was performed by the Rand Corporation. They concluded that short-term chiropractic therapy was beneficial for uncomplicated joint problems without serious symptoms, such as severe leg pain or a herniated disk. This research also concluded that you should see results within the first month of care. If you find that chiropractic therapy aggravates your condition or is not helping, stop seeing the chiropractor and get a second opinion. Although serious side effects from spinal manipulation are rare, they do occur. It has been estimated that a stroke can occur once every 500,000 to 2,000,000 manipulations. If you have osteoporosis, cancer or any serious illness, only see a chiropractor who uses the most gentle types of manipulations and use your chiropractor as an adjunct to traditional medical care.

HOMEOPATHY—LIKE CURES LIKE

The basic principle of homeopathy is that "like cures like." This system of therapy was developed by Samuel Hahnemann. He experimented with the physiological reactions caused by ingesting certain foods and chemicals. He theorizes and in some cases has documented that prescribing a small amount of a substance can sometimes relieve adverse symptoms caused by ingesting large amounts of that same substance. Vaccines use a similar process. Vaccines are often a weakened virus or bacteria which, when injected into the body, help the body mount a defense against disease. In a similar way, homeopathy claims that a minute dose of the same thing that, in larger doses, would produce your symptoms, will cure it.

The *British Medical Journal* suggests that homeopathic remedies may help conditions such as diarrhea, asthma, hay fever, the flu and chronic headaches. However, because homeopathy is still new and controversial, it should not be the treatment of choice for a serious illness unless you have first checked with your physician.

MASSAGE THERAPY—TOUCH THERAPY

Not only is massage therapy part of almost every healing tradition, it is also found in health spas, athletic clubs and many health care clinics. Massage can improve circulation, reduce swelling, improve range of motion and eliminate tight, spastic muscles. It is especially effective with mild to moderate back and neck pain which is muscular in origin. It is not appropriate for serious spinal injury unless you have already consulted with your physician. However, if you have already tried traditional medical care for your problem, massage may be a reasonable alternative, especially if you suspect tight muscles are the culprit.

There are many styles of massage, some gentler and more relaxing, others stronger and more probing which are termed *deep tissue*. Always start with the gentler therapy first, choosing deeper massage if the gentler version has not aggravated your condition. Avoid massage therapy if you have a serious infection, cancer or some other type of serious disease as massage can actually spread the disease.

NATUROPATHY—THE NATURE DOCS

Naturopathic physicians attend one of a handful of four-year natural medicine colleges earning the right to call themselves Doctors of Naturopathy. Most naturopaths are well-trained in diagnosis and use herbal medicine, nutrition and homeopathy to treat illness. Some naturopaths even use acupuncture, spinal manipulation and massage. Many states license naturopaths, and although they are most popular in the northwestern United States, they are rapidly gaining acceptance in other areas as well. Naturopaths use many standard medical lab tests and diagnostic methods and can effectively treat many types of health problems. Because their therapies do not use drugs, you can feel confident that this type of therapy is reasonably safe.

However, be cautious of any prescription for large doses of vitamins or a detoxification program involving any severe dietary practice.

Also, be certain that your naturopath has graduated from an accredited college. Unfortunately, there are fly-by-night diploma mills that provide N.D. degrees through simple correspondence courses.

PSYCHOTHERAPY

Psychiatrists, psychologists, marriage and family counselors—even your local minister or rabbi can provide psychotherapy. An hour or two of talking about your problems with some professional guidance can be quite valuable.

Most psychotherapists have received two to four years of post-graduate academic training with additional hours of supervised clinical practice. Although psychotherapy has been shown to be extremely effective with many kinds of psychological problems, such as anxiety and depression, it does have its limits. Some conditions, such as bi-polar disorder (manic-depression), are biochemical in nature and require a balancing of the faulty chemistry. If you have tried five sessions of psychotherapy with a qualified practitioner and have experienced no improvement, talk to your doctor. You may need to have your physician or a psychiatrist prescribe medication to alleviate your condition, or you may need to look for a mental health professional experienced in handling your problem.

:60 SECOND COMPLIMENTARY MEDICINE SUMMARY

- Because medical doctors have the broadest access to diagnostic tools, they should be the first people you turn to for expert advice.
- Acupuncturists believe that the acupuncture needles and the use of herbal medicine can modify your life force helping to remedy many illnesses.
- Chiropractors can provide manipulation, massage and exercise therapy to help alleviate some conditions.
- Homeopathy claims that a minute dose of the same substance that would, in larger doses, produce your symptoms, will cure them.
- Massage therapy is touted as a cure for almost all of life's ills and may be a reasonable alternative for many conditions which are muscular in origin.
- Naturopathy involves the use of herbal medicine, nutrition, homeopathy, acupuncture, spinal manipulation and massage.
- Talking about your problems with a variety of professionals can be quite helpful.

Chapter 24

REJUVENATION—WHERE DO I START? WHEN AM I DONE?

:60 Second Affirmation:
"Each day I experience my life unfolding."

Chris began studying for his master's in business administration when he was twenty years old. After completing his studies, he became a day trader in the stock market, where he was able to earn a comfortable living, eventually developing a portfolio worth more than one million dollars. But with each month, he became more tired.

He went to his doctor complaining of fatigue, occasional dizziness, headaches and a lack of appetite. Although he knew that excessive stress, smoking cigarettes and eating fast food were unhealthy, he did not have the time or discipline to change all his bad habits.

This went on for months until he finally lacked the stamina to get out of bed. A return visit to the doctor confirmed that he had Lyme disease. The treatment was an immediate course of antibiotics. After four weeks of medication, he felt partially recovered. He could get out of bed but still lacked the energy he felt prior to becoming ill. Chris then came to me for help. He explained that he was willing to make changes but felt that he lacked the discipline to do so. He did not know where to start.

I explained to him that, although he desired to make drastic changes in his lifestyle, small, steady improvements were more lasting. And the most fundamental lifestyle components that needed to be changed were his poor diet and lack of exercise.

He began the :60 Second Rejuvenation Strategy diet, primarily subsisting on fresh fruits, vegetables and whole grains, supplemented with lean fish and chicken. I even allowed him to eat eggs, nuts, seeds and some red meat. He was to avoid all other food until he began to feel better. I insisted that he stop eating all fast food, except for one visit to his favorite fast food restaurant each week. Because the :60 Second Rejuvenation Strategy diet allows one to eat a wide variety of foods, he did not find the diet difficult.

Two weeks later, I asked him to take a multivitamin and mineral supplement each day with some strengthening herbs including siberian ginseng and echinacea. The following month, I asked him to walk for fifteen to thirty minutes each day and to begin to drink green or black tea at least once each day instead of coffee. I continued to slowly introduce healthier habits into Chris's previously sedentary, unhealthy lifestyle. After six months he had lost fifteen pounds, had his strength back and was again excelling in his career. I did not ask him to stop smoking yet because I knew that it would be too difficult a task. It was easy to ask him to eat healthier, take supplements and engage in regular exercise.

When I felt it was time, I referred Chris to a physician who specialized in addiction. After two months on a nicotine patch, supplemented by acupuncture and massage, he was free of his nicotine addiction. Luckily, his physician also referred him to a meditation course sponsored by the local hospital. Chris was again making a lot of money and now had the good health to enjoy it. By using principles of the :60 Second Rejuvenation Strategy, he was able to transform his life one step at a time.

POSITIVE REINFORCEMENT

Before studying natural therapies, I was a learning disabilities specialist. My job was to identify children who were failing in school, properly evaluate them and improve their academic and social skills. I worked with some children that were difficult to help. One thing I learned was the power of positive reinforcement. Just as Pavlov's dogs would salivate at the first sight of a juicy steak, people are encouraged and uplifted by compliments, praise and social reward.

I learned that changing a child's behavior required two things:

1. Breaking all tasks into small, easy to learn steps.
2. Providing regular systematic rewards with only occasional criticism and punishment.

Small steps are easier to accomplish and most of those steps should be pleasurable. Even the legendary psychoanalyst, Sigmund Freud, taught that our life is driven by a search for pleasure and reward.

ONE STEP AT A TIME

Don't try to radically change your life in one week. Think of improved health and spiritual well-being as a lifelong process. Each day try to focus on one small bad habit which you would like to eliminate and one good habit you want to initiate. Feel good about any changes and improvements you have already made. To "catch yourself doin' good" you must do these things:

1. Decide which behavior you want to change.
2. Make the smallest change possible.
3. Be consistent in implementing the change.
4. If you falter, begin again.

DON'T STOP, JUST START

Attempting to drastically change or completely stop bad habits will only destine you for failure. It is far easier to add a new behavior than it is to stop a lifelong habit. Merely adding a salad and a piece of fruit everyday to your diet could improve the quality of your life and reduce your risk of cancer, heart disease and other illnesses significantly.

As we approach the year 2000, the life expectancy at birth is around eighty years. If you avoid smoking, heavy alcohol consumption, eat a balanced diet and exercise moderately, you can expect to live to be eighty or ninety years old. More importantly, if you are or when you are sixty, you could look forward to twenty to thirty years of healthy, prosperous living. Make the most of these years by beginning a healthy lifestyle today and implementing the *:60 Second Rejuvenation Strategy* one step at a time.

:60 SECOND SYMPTOM SUBSTITUTION

Another excellent method to improve your life is to substitute one behavior for another. Choose any unhealthy behavior and make it just a little bit healthier. Here are a few suggestions for small steps that you can take:

1. If you love a huge bowl of ice cream, laden with saturated fat and artery-clogging cholesterol, try an alternative. You could try a low-fat ice cream, non-fat frozen yogurt or sorbet. Add a few fresh berries to the top of your low-fat treat instead of hot fudge, nuts and whipped cream, and you have a dessert that is far healthier and could actually reduce your risk of cancer and heart disease.
2. If you park your car one block from work, try parking two or three blocks away in the future.
3. If you smoke, try reducing the number of cigarettes you have each week and smoke a lower tar and nicotine version.
4. If you frequently eat a large steak for dinner, try eating a leaner and smaller cut.
5. Forget that candy bar after lunch. Try a piece of fruit instead.
6. Don't sit in front of your computer for three or four hours without a break. Make an effort to stand up every twenty to thirty minutes.
7. Cut out one cup of coffee and try drinking a glass of spring water or green or black tea.
8. Get up in the morning five minutes earlier and perform a few stretching exercises or walk around the block before getting in your car and going to work.
9. Practice meditation or the chest-belly-exhale technique on arising or before going to sleep.
10. Go to bed at the same time every night, especially on the weekend.
11. Start taking a multivitamin, multimineral supplement on a regular basis.
12. Leave your house for any appointment one to two minutes early so that you can relax and enjoy a stress-free trip.

Each time you fail to achieve your larger goal you will be less willing to try to change, but small changes are easier to implement and can make a big difference. Just take small meaningful steps in the right direction.

OKAY, BUT WHERE DO I START?

There are many ways to begin your *:60 Second Rejuvenation Strategy.* Try meditating for :60 seconds and see what comes to mind. Think about yourself. What is the one behavior that makes you feel most uncomfortable or that bothers you the most? Perhaps that is where you should start. Now think of an another behavior that also needs improving. Which of these two behaviors would be the easiest to modify? Be certain that the first behavior you choose to try to change is the easier one. The :60 *Second Rejuvenation Strategy* is a simple process to follow and is based upon healthy habits which are natural, therefore it should be relatively easy to integrate into your life. However, any change may be difficult to implement for some individuals.

DIET—THE BASICS

Eat plenty of fruits and vegetables every day; at least five servings or fifty percent of your diet. Remember that a salad can count as two or three servings if it is a mixture of different vegetables. Regularly snack on fruit and try throwing some sliced banana or fresh berries on your next dessert. Supplement these fruits and vegetables with a wide variety of protein sources—try eating one serving per day of either lean fish or chicken, eggs, nuts, dairy products and beans or tofu instead of something high in fat like a fast food hamburger. Eat one to two servings of each of these valuable high-protein foods each week and avoid fatty beef or pork except on rare, special occasions.

Drink lots of liquid, especially spring or filtered water and green tea. Although heavy consumption should be avoided, according to recent studies, one to two cups of coffee or alcohol each day poses no health hazard.

EXERCISE

Try to perform at least thirty minutes of cardiovascular exercise, three times each week. Walking, swimming and bicycling are all ideal exercises because they are low-impact. To increase flexibility, perform the :60 *Second Rejuvenation Strategy's* stretching exercises regularly and try taking a beginning yoga or tai chi class at least once a week. Stretching a few minutes per day, each day, will eventually produce dramatic results. To improve your strength, go to the gym two or three times a week and start a general weight training program. If a gym is inconvenient or too costly, you can purchase a set of one- to two-pound dumbbells and ankle weights at a sporting goods store and perform some simple strengthening exercises at home.

MEDITATION AND PRAYER

Regular prayer and meditation will teach you to focus your mind, diverting it from chatter. Try meditating or praying for five minutes each day or just close your eyes :60 seconds a few times each day and use the belly-chest-exhale technique.

Always think positive. When you drive your car, you steer around debris and potholes. Try driving your mind around negative thoughts. Focus on your family, good friends, things you love to do or spiritual ideals. Try reading the Bible or an inspirational book of affirmations and choose friends who you find spiritually uplifting.

SLEEP

Try going to sleep and waking up at approximately the same time each day, particularly on the weekend when most of us would like to stay up late and sleep in late. Be certain that your bed and pillow are comfortable and your room is the proper temperature. Avoid stimulating activity, food and drink late in the evening. Avoid bright lights as the evening progresses.

TRANSPORTATION

Make sure your driver's seat is comfortable. If you are taking a long trip, remember to stop periodically to get out and stretch. When you are able, try walking more and driving less. For example, vary your morning commute by taking the subway, using your bicycle or taking a bus once in awhile. Avoiding rush hour traffic in your car may help you to feel less stressed.

THE POSTURE PRINCIPLE

Proper body alignment will rejuvenate your mind, body and spirit. Practice finding the neutral posture position many times during the day to reduce stress and increase your sense of well-being.

YOUR FIVE STRESS ZONES

Pay attention to each stress zone throughout the day. Notice where you hold tension. Use the :60 second techniques in this book to relieve tension in these important areas. If you cannot release stress in a particular region, seek out the help of a trained professional. Your doctor, a massage therapist, an acupuncturist, a physical therapist or a chiropractor can all be helpful when you have areas of chronic tension.

SENSUALITY VS. SEXUALITY

Remember, a sensual life is very important. It is even more important than a sexual life. Comfortable clothing, a good massage, masturbation, even dancing can all provoke sensual pleasure and the calming, relaxing effect it creates. It is important that you enjoy your life and your body whatever your age. Healthy thoughts and healthy sexuality are both natural outgrowths of this way of living.

COMPLIMENTARY MEDICINE

Herbal remedies, acupuncture, chiropractic, homeopathy and naturopathy are all gentle therapies. Some have been used for hundreds, even thousands, of years. Read literature on complimentary medicine and seek out a qualified practitioner to help you in your *:60 Second Rejuvenation Strategy.*

PUTTING IT ALL TOGETHER

A diet comprised of mostly natural foods, regular gentle exercise, a calm mind, proper posture and spiritual development can be the basis to a healthy long life. Remember that the principles of the *:60 Second Rejuvenation Strategy* are based upon the behaviors of our ancient ancestors, are more natural than artificial diets or fad exercise routines and involve real changes that will last a lifetime. Refer back to the *:60 Second Rejuvenation Strategy* whenever you have questions about healthy living.

:60 SECOND LIFELONG HEALTH SUMMARY

- Think of improved health and spiritual well-being as a lifelong process.
- Decide which one behavior you want to change first, make the smallest change possible, be consistent and begin again if you falter.
- Adding a new behavior is far easier than trying to stop a life-long habit.

- Substitute one behavior for another; take any behavior and make it just a little bit healthier.
- Proper diet, regular exercise, meditation and prayer, adequate and restful sleep, transportation alternatives, correct posture, the five stress zones, sensuality and sexuality and complimentary medicine are all integral considerations of the :60 Second Rejuvenation Strategy.

:60 SECOND HEALTH AND NUTRITION QUIZ

Do you have a healthy concept of diet and nutrition? Below you will find some common behaviors and beliefs regarding health and nutrition. Read each statement carefully. If you think it is true for you, place a mark in the "true" column. If you feel it does not apply to you, place a mark in the "false" column. There is a scoring section at the end of the quiz to give you an idea of how healthy your diet is.

	True	False
1. I drink at least six cups of water each day.	____	____
2. The water I drink is bottled or filtered.	____	____
3. When making a sandwich, I use whole-grain bread.	____	____
4. I choose brown rice over white.	____	____
5. I supplement my diet with a high-quality multivitamin.	____	____
6. When I crave ice cream, I choose a low-fat variety or frozen yogurt.	____	____
7. I frequently choose fish or poultry over beef and pork.	____	____
8. I supplement my diet with beans, tofu, legumes and nuts	____	____
9. I usually bake, roast or broil my food instead of frying it.	____	____
10. When I do fry foods, I use unsaturated oils such as olive and canola.	____	____
11. I drink at least one cup of green or black tea each day.	____	____
12. I eat at least five servings of fruits and vegetables each day.	____	____
13. I only use non-fat or low-fat dairy products.	____	____

	True	False
14. I usually have at least one piece of fruit with breakfast.	___	___
15. Pasta is not a major part of my diet.	___	___
16. When I crave sweets, I reach for a piece of fruit.	___	___
17. I occasionally eat eggs with breakfast.	___	___
18. I always have fresh fruits and vegetables available in my home.	___	___
19. I drink soda, wine and coffee in moderation.	___	___
20. Even when dieting, I make sure I consume some fat.	___	___
21. I only drink one to two cups of coffee per day.	___	___
22. I take echinacea, goldenseal or garlic when I start to get a cold or the flu.	___	___
23. I avoid foods high in preservatives or artificial flavors or colorings.	___	___
24. I do not eat large meals or drink caffeinated beverages late in the day.	___	___
25. Processed foods make up a small portion of my diet.	___	___
26. When eating a meal, I do not engage in any other activities.	___	___
27. I am aware of the way my body reacts after I eat certain foods.	___	___
28. I always follow a cup of coffee with a glass of water.	___	___
29. Sometimes I take natural remedies instead of medication.	___	___
30. Instead of eating when I need an energy boost, I exercise.	___	___

Scoring: Score one point for each "true" answer.

20-30 "true" answers: Your nutritional habits are very healthy! Continue eating well and maintaining your health diet.

10-20 "true" answers: You have a relatively healthy diet, but need to increase your nutritional awareness. Try learning more about nutrition and implementing small improvements (like those described in the *:60 Second Rejuvenation Strategy*) in your dietary regimen.

0-10 "true" answers: You need to learn much more about good nutrition and make an effort to apply what you learned from the *:60 Second Rejuvenation Strategy*. Ask your doctor or nutritionist for advice on how to improve your dietary habits. Go over the *:60 Second Rejuvenation Strategy* again!

:60 SECOND MENTAL AND PHYSICAL WELL-BEING QUIZ

How healthy is your lifestyle? Below you will find some common behaviors and beliefs regarding physical and mental health and wellness. Read each statement carefully. If you think it is true for you, place a mark in the "true" column. If you feel it does not apply to you, place a mark in the "false" column. There is a scoring section at the end of the quiz to give you an idea of how healthy you are.

	True	False
1. When I am at work I frequently get up from my desk and stretch.	_____	_____
2. I always make sure my car seat is comfortable before I begin a long drive.	_____	_____
3. I do not slouch when I am sitting or standing.	_____	_____
4. If I realize I am breathing shallowly, I consciously take deep, slow breaths.	_____	_____
5. When my muscles become tense, I immediately stretch and relax them.	_____	_____
6. I meditate to calm my mind.	_____	_____
7. When I sit for long periods of time, I continually readjust my posture.	_____	_____
8. At home, I sit in a recliner or with my back slightly reclined.	_____	_____
9. I exercise on a regular basis (at least three times per week).	_____	_____
10. I always stretch before engaging in physical activities.	_____	_____
11. Even in stressful situations, I try to keep my muscles relaxed.	_____	_____
12. I do not engage in dangerous sports in which I could be seriously injured.	_____	_____

	True	False
13. When I notice I am slouching, I immediately improve my posture.	____	____
14. When on the phone, I keep my neck straight.	____	____
15. When reading, I keep my book at eye-level.	____	____
16. I never sleep on my stomach.	____	____
17. At work, my desk or the area I work in is set up so that I am comfortable.	____	____
18. I consult my doctor when I have a medical problem of a serious nature.	____	____
19. I breathe deeply and slowly to help myself relax.	____	____
20. I have used alternative treatments for physical ailments.	____	____
21. During long drives, I stop frequently to stretch.	____	____
22. I stretch when I wake up in the morning and before I go to sleep at night.	____	____
23. I express anger and other emotions in healthy ways.	____	____
24. When I sleep, my pillow keeps my head and neck properly supported.	____	____
25. I make decisions quickly instead of worrying about them.	____	____
26. I enjoy a healthy and loving sexual relationship.	____	____
27. I engage in exercises or activities that help me relieve stress.	____	____
28. When I am nervous or under pressure at work, I remain calm and focused.	____	____
29. I unwind and clear my mind before I go to bed.	____	____
30. I go to sleep at the same time every night.	____	____

Scoring: Score one point for each "true" answer.

20-30 "true" answers: You are very healthy physically, mentally and spiritually! Continue to relieve stress and rejuvenate your mind and body through exercise, stretching regimens and meditation.

10-20 "true" answers: You have a relatively healthy lifestyle, but need to learn more about activities that alleviate stress and improve physical and mental well-being. Increase your knowledge of healthy living and implement more of the :60 Second Rejuvenation Strategies into your daily life.

0-10 "true" answers: You need to learn much more about mental, spiritual and physical well-being and make an effort to apply what you learned from the :60 Second Rejuvenation Strategy. Consult your doctor for advice on how to improve your lifestyle. See a naturopathic physician, join a gym or try yoga or meditation. Read the :60 Second Rejuvenation Strategy again!

APPENDIX

Exercises Utilizing the Thera-Cane

NECK

FOR ALL NECK POSITIONS.
Lean neck into ball,
hands & Cane remain still.

Move neck side to side &
up & down for pressure.

Also try these in
the supine position.
Elevate head with pillows.

Use your fingers for
the front and side of
neck muscles.

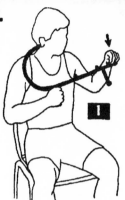

#1 NECK

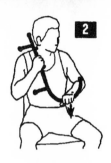

#5 NECK

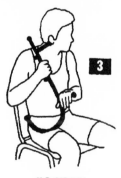

#3 NECK

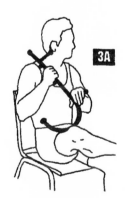

Cross legs to
adjust position.

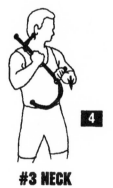

#3 NECK

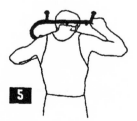

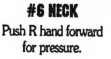

#6 NECK
Push R hand forward
for pressure.

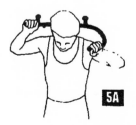

SHOULDERS

FOR ALL SHOULDER POSITIONS.

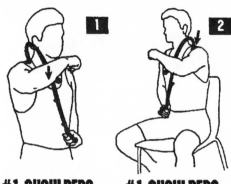

#1 SHOULDERS

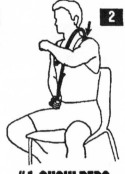

#1 SHOULDERS

Push down in the direction of the arrows for pressure.

Move upper arms back & forth 1-2 inches for cross friction massage.

Keep arms in close to side.

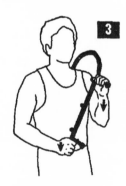

#1 SHOULDERS

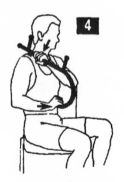

#5 SHOULDERS

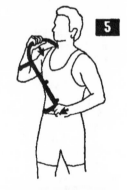

#1 SHOULDERS

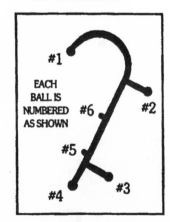

EACH BALL IS NUMBERED AS SHOWN

#1 #6 #2 #5 #4 #3

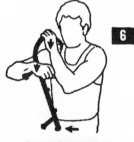

#1 SHOULDERS
Cane leans against front of leg.

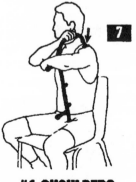

#1 SHOULDERS

BACK

Loop over L shoulder to work on R shoulder blade.

#1 UPPER BACK
Push L hand downward then push R hand forward 1-2 inches for pressure.

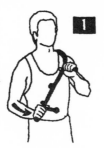 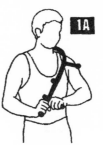 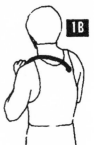

Best back position for big bodies

Alternate hand position.

Rotate R shoulder blade forward for hard to get points.

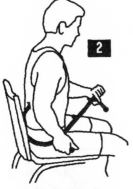

#1 LOW BACK
Stabilize against chair & lean into ball.

Keep back & buttocks 2-3 inches from the back of the chair.

Cane held off to side.

Move side to side for cross friction massage.

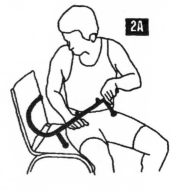

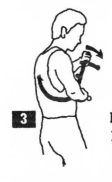

#1 UPPER & MID BACK
Tilt Cane upward for best leverage.
Push L hand downward 1-2 inches for pressure.
R arm remains still.

#1 LOW BACK
Lean back in chair directly against the ball.

 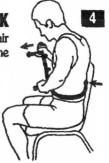

Push R hand outward 1-2 inches for pressure, then move upper body side to side for cross friction massage.

BACK

#6 UPPER & MID BACK
Push R arm forward for pressure.

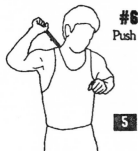

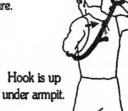
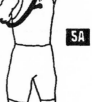

Hook is up
under armpit.

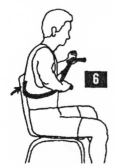
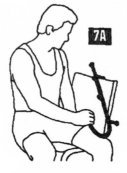
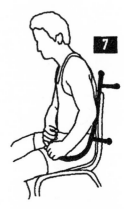

#1 MID BACK
Lean back in chair
directly against ball.
Keep R arm locked
in place.

Stabilize against chair
& lean into ball.
Move side to side
for cross friction massage.

#5 UPPER BACK

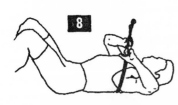
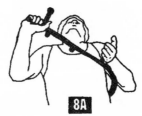

#1 BACK
Elevate your head with some pillows.

Vary hand grip
open palm is easy.

The supine position is the most versatile.
experiment on your own!

BIBLIOGRAPHY

Balch, James F. *Prescription for Nutritional Healing: A Practical A-Z Reference to Drug-Free Remedies Using Vitamins, Minerals, Herbs and Food Supplements.* New York: Avery Publishing Group Inc., 1996.

Cranz, Galen. *The Chair: Rethinking Culture, Body, and Design.* New York: W.W. Norton & Company, 1998.

Crawford, Michael and David Marsh. *Nutrition And Evolution: Food in Evolution and the Future.* Connecticut: Keats Publishing, Inc., 1995.

Dement, William. *The Promise of Sleep.* New York: Random House, 1999.

DesMaisons, Kathleen. *Potatoes Not Prozac: A Natural Seven-Step Dietary Plan to Stabilize the Level of Sugar in Your Blood, Control Your Cravings, and Lose Weight.* New York: Simon & Schuster, 1998.

Folline, Stefania and Carol Orlock. *Know Your Body Clock.* New York: Citadel Press, 1995.

Gogoghian, Shoto and Dan Georgakas. *The Methuselah Factors: Learning From the World's Longest Living People.* Illinois: Academy Chicago Publishers, 1995.

Johns, Timothy. *The Origins Of Human Diet & Medicine: Chemical Ecology (Arizona Studies in Human Ecology).* Tucson: The University Of Arizona Press, 1996.

Lamrimpa, Gen. *Calming The Mind: Tibetan Buddhist Teachings on the Cultivation of Meditative Quiescence.* Edited by Hart Sprager. New York: Snow Lion Publications, 1992.

Netzer, Corinne T. *The Complete Book Of Food Counts.* 4th Ed. New York: Dell Publishing, 1997.

Weiss, Rudolf F. *Herbal Medicine.* England: Beaconsfield Publishers Ltd., AB Arcanum, 1988.

Articles

Ames, Bruce N. "The Causes and Prevention of Cancer" *Biotherapy* 11, nos. 2-3 (1998): 205-20.

Ames, Bruce N. "Micronutrients Prevent and Delay Aging." *Toxicology Letter* 102-103 (December 1998): 5-18.

Bailey, D.M. "Blood Lipid and Lipoprotein Concentration in Active, Sedentary, Healthy, and Diseased Men." *Journal of Cardiovascular Risk* 5, nos. 5-6 (October-December 1998): 309-312.

Barefoot, J. "Trust, Health and Longevity." *Journal of Behavioral Medicine* 21, no. 6 (December 1998): 517-26.

Bass, C. "Frequent Attenders Without Organic Disease in a Gastroenterology Clinic." *General Hospital Psychiatry* 21, no. 1 (January-February 1999): 30-1.

Bortz, W.M. "Physical Fitness, Aging and Sexuality." *Western Journal of Medicine* 170, no. 3 (March 1997): 167-9.

Bowman Gray School of Medicine. "Assessing the Observed Relationship Between Low Cholesterol and Violence-related Mortality." *Annals of New York Academy of Science* 836 (29 December 1997): 57-80.

Caygill, C.P. "Relationship Between the Intake of High Fiber Foods and the Risks of Cancer." *European Journal of Cancer Prevention* 7, Suppl. 2 (May 1998): S11-7.

Center for Human Nutrition. "Alterations in Mood After Changing to a Low-fat Diet." *British Journal of Nutrition* 79, no. 1 (January 1998): 23-30.

Cohen, S. "Psychological Stress and Susceptibility to the Common Cold." *New England Journal of Medicine* 325, no. 9 (29 August 1991): 606-12.

Davis, Clara and D.M. Davis. "Results of the Self-selection of Diets of Young Children." *Canadian Medical Association Journal* 41 (1939): 257-61.

DeStefani, E. "Diet and Cancer of the Upper Digestive Tract." *Oral Oncology* 35, no. 1 (January 1999): 17-21.

"Effects of Eating Behavior on Mood: A Review of the Literature." *International Journal of Eating Disorders* 14, no. 2 (September 1993): 171-83.

Elmst, S. "Dietary Patterns in High and Low Consumers of Meat in a Swedish Cohort Study." *Appetite* 32, no. 2 (April 1999): 191-206.

The Framingham Study. "Serum Cholesterol, Lipoproteins, and the Risk of Coronary Heart Disease." *Annals of Internal Medicine* 74, no. 1 (January 1971): 1-12.

Herbert, J.R. "The Effect of Dietary Exposures on Recurrence and Mortality in Early Stage Breast Cancer." *Breast Cancer Research and Treatment* 51, no. 1 (September 1998): 17-28.

Hicks, R.A. "The Incidence of Sleep Problems Among Type A and Type B College Students: Changes Over a Ten-Year Period (1982-1992)." *Perceptual and Motor Skills* 75, no. 3, pt. 1 (December 1992): 746.

Hollman, P.C. "Tea Flavinoids in Cardiovascular Disease and Cancer Epidemiology." *Proceedings of The Society of Experimental Biology and Medicine* (University of Pennsylvania) 220, no. 4 (April 1999): 198-202.

Hsieh, C.C. "Predictors of Sex Hormone Levels Among the Elderly." *Journal of Clinical Epidemiology* 51, no. 10 (October 1998): 837-41.

Hu, F.B. "A Prospective Study on Egg Consumption and Risk of Cardiovascular Disease in Men and Women." *Journal of the American Medical Association* 28, no. 15 (21 April 1999): 1387-94.

Hurwitz, E.L. "Manipulation and Mobilization of the Cervical Spine: A Systematic Review of the Literature." *Spine* 21, no. 15 (1 August 1996): 1746-59.

Jacobs, D.R, "Is Whole Grain Intake Associated With Total and Cause Specific Death Rates in Older Women." *American Journal of Public Health* 89, no. 3 (March 1999): 322-9.

Jewett, Stephen. "Longevity and the Longevity Syndrome." *The Gerontologist* 12, no. 1 (Spring 1973): 91-99.

Kampman, E. "Meat Consumption, Genetic Susceptibility and Colon Cancer Risk." *Cancer Epidemiology Biomarkers and Prevention* 8, no. 1 (January 1999): 15-24.

Kleijnen, J. "Commissioning Complementary Medicine. Homeopathic Hospitals Have Unique Skill." *British Medical Journal* 1, no. 6174 (19 May 1979): 1354-5.

Kleiner, S.M. "Water: An Essential But Overlooked Nutrient." *Journal of the American Dietetics Association* 99, no. 2 (February 1999): 200-6.

Levi, F. "Food Groups and the Risk of Oral and Pharyngeal Cancer." *International Journal of Cancer* 77, no. 5 (31 August 1998): 705-9.

Levi, F. "Food Groups and Colorectal Cancer Risk." *British Journal of Cancer* 79, nos. 7-8 (March 1999): 1287-7.

McCrory, M.A. "Dietary Variety Within Food Groups: Association with Energy Intake and Body Fatness in Men and Women." *American Journal of Clinical Nutrition* 69, no. 3 (March 1999): 440-7.

Mills, James. "Prevention, Detection, Evaluation and Treatment of High Blood Pressure." Sixth Report of the NIH Joint National Committee, Washington, DC, NIH Publication 98-4080, November 1997.

"Mood Modulation by Food: An Exploration of Affect and Cravings on 'Chocolate Addicts'." *British Journal of Psychology* 34, pt. 1 (February 1995): 129-38.

Morin, C.M. "Nonpharmacological Treatment of Late-life Insomnia." *Journal of Psychosomatic Research* 46, no. 2 (February 1999): 103-16.

Munoz, M. "Diet That Prevents Cancer." *International Journal of Cancer* 11, Suppl. (1998): 85-9.

National Cancer Institute. "Pesticides and Childhood Cancer." *Environmental Health Perspectives* 106, no. 3 (June 1998): 893-908.

Nygaard, I. "Thirst at Work: an Occupation Hazard?" *International Urological Journal* 8, no. 6 (1997): 340-343, 20.

Olive, M.F. "Compensatory Sleep Responses to Wakefulness Induced by the Dopamine Autoreceptor Antagonist." *Journal of Pharmacology and Experimental Therapeutics* 285, no. 3 (June 1998): 1073-83.

"Pain Perception in Patients with Eating Disorders." *Psychosomatic Medicine* (University of Sheffield) 52, no. 6 (November-December 1990): 673-82.

"Paleolithic Nutrition. A Consideration of its Nature and Current Implications." *New England Journal of Medicine* 312, no. 5 (31 January 1985): 283-9.

Petridou, E. "Diet During Pregnancy and the Risk of Cerebral Palsy." *British Journal of Nutrition* 79, no. 5 (May 1998): 405-12.

Pritikin, Nathan. "The Pritikin Diet." *Journal of the American Medical Association* 251, no. 9 (2 March 1984): 1160-1.

"Proceedings of the Second Annual International Scientific Symposium on Tea and Human Health." Washington, DC, 14 September 1998.

"Reversing Heart Disease Through Diet, Exercise and Stress Management: An Interview with Dr. Dean Ornish." *Journal of the American Dietetics Association* 91, no. 2 (February 1991): 162-5.

Rossignol, A.M. "Caffeine-containing Beverages, Total Fluid Consumption and Premenstrual Syndrome." *American Journal of Public Health* 80, no. 9 (September 1990): 1106-10.

Roquejo, A.M. "The Age at Which Meat is First Introduced into the Diet." *International Journal of Vitamin and Nutritional Research* 69, no. 2 (March 1999): 127-31.

Sponheimer, M. "Isotopic Evidence for the Diet of an Early Hominid." *Science* 283, no. 5400 (15 January 1999): 368-70.

Stout, N.R. "A Review of Water Balance in Aging in Health and Disease." *Gerontology* 45, no. 2 (1999): 61-6.

Tsutsumi, T. "Comparison of High and Moderate Intensity of Strength Training on Mood and Anxiety on Older Adults." *Perceptual and Motor Skills* 87, no. 3, pt. 1 (December 1998): 1003-11.

Videman, T. "Lumbar Spinal Pathology in Cadaveric Material in Relation to History of Back Pain, Occupation and Physical Loading." *Spine* 15, no. 8 (August 1990): 728-40.

Wahlqvist, M.L. "Aging, Food, Culture and Health." *Southeast Asian Journal of Tropical Medicine and Public Health* 28, suppl. 2 (1997): 100-12.

Zheng, W. "Well Done Meat Intake and the Risk of Breast Cancer." *Journal of The National Cancer Institute* 90, no. 22 (18 November 1998): 1724-9.